Heirloom Treasures
Recipes
From
Granny Ruth
And
Granny Betty

Heirloom Treasures:

Recipes from Granny Ruth and Granny Betty

Explore the cherished culinary legacies of two remarkable women with "Heirloom Treasures: Recipes from Granny Ruth and Granny Betty." This cookbook is a heartfelt tribute to the timeless recipes of two grandmothers whose kitchens were the heart of their homes.

Granny Ruth and Granny Betty have left behind a treasure trove of recipes, lovingly preserved and compiled. Their culinary creations are a testament to family, love, and tradition. This collection features beautifully photographed dishes, each telling a story of family gatherings, holidays, and everyday home-cooked meals. Alongside the images, you'll find anecdotes that bring these recipes to life, offering a glimpse into the warmth of their kitchens.

You'll also find scanned images of handwritten recipes, preserving the personal touch of Granny Ruth and Granny Betty. These recipes are pieces of history passed down through generations. For ease of use, many recipes have been meticulously typed out, ensuring you can recreate these beloved dishes with confidence.

"Heirloom Treasures" is more than just a cookbook; it's a family heirloom. Whether you're an experienced cook or a kitchen novice, this collection invites you to savor the flavors of the past and create new memories. Enjoy the warmth, love, and deliciousness shared through these timeless recipes.

1½ cups Judges 4:19 <u>milk</u>
Seasoning. II Chronicles 9:9 <u>Spices</u>
Follow the directions of Solomon
for bringing up a Child Proverbs
23:14

Old Testament Cake

4½ Cups I Kings 4:22 _flour_
1 - Cup Judges 5:25 (last clause) _Butter_
2 - Cups Jeremiah 6:20 _Sugar_
2 - Cups I Samuel 30:12 _Raisins_
2 - Cups Nahum 3:12 _figs_
2 - Cups Numbers 17:8 _Almonds_
2 - Tablespoons I Samuel 14:25 _honey_
1 - Pinch Leviticus 2:13 _Salt_
6 - Jeremiah 17:11 _Eggs_

$100 Chocolate Cake

½ cup butter
2 cups sugar
4 oz (4 squares Chocolate unsweetened)
2 eggs
1½ cups sweet milk
2 cups flour
2 tsp. Baking powder
2 " Vanilla
1 cup Nuts   walnuts or other kinds

Cream butter + Sugar. add melted Chocolate
+ beaten eggs. sift dry ingredients
add) alternately with milk add Vanilla + Nuts
Bake in ~~Rep one~~ lope pan for 45 minutes at 350

Icing

½ cup butter   1 pinch salt
2 oz Chocolate   1 tsp Vanilla
1 Egg   1" lemon juice
1½ Cups powdered Sugar 1 cup nuts

Melt butter + Cho together. Add beaten Eggs
Sugar salt Vanilla + lemon juice
Mix in Nuts or sprinkle on top

Strawberry Pie

1 Cup Sugar
1 Cup water
3 tablespoons Cornstarch
Cook until thickens
Remove from heat + add 3
teaspoons of Strawberry Jello.
Powder form + two or three
drops of Red Cake Coloring + pinch
of Salt. Pour half of filling in
pie shell. add layer of fresh
strawberries then rest of filling.
top with Whip Cream

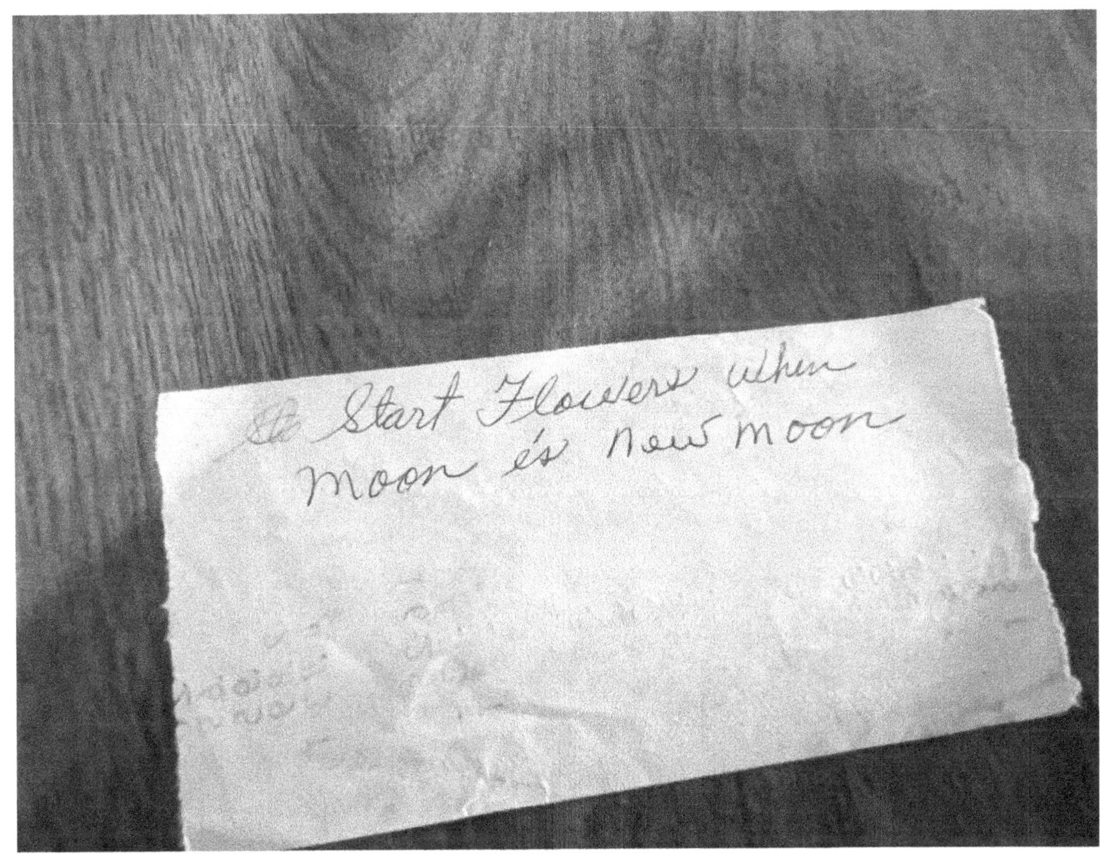
Start Flowers when
Moon is New moon

"30 Day Friendship Cake"

<u>Do not cover</u> this tightly. Just lay something on <u>Top</u>

1 - large can of peaches sliced up and put in the starter liquid. Stir each day for 10 days.

Add -

2½ cups sugar and 1 large can undrained Crushed pineapple. Stir each day for 10 days

Then Add -

3 - 9oz marchino Cherries (drained) diced & stir each day for 10 more days.

Makes 3 cakes.

For each Cake

1 - box yellow or lemon cake mix (I used lemon)

1 - box instant vanilla pudding (I used Butter Pecan)

¾ - Cup oil   2 Cups brewed fruit

4 - eggs   1 - Cup flaked Coconut

1 - Cup nuts

1 - Cup raisins (optional)

Bake in bundt pan or regular cake pans for 45 to 1 hr 350 degrees

It freezes well, but don't put icing on it before freezing.

You might think the fruit is ruined but just keeping stirring its okay

Cream butter & shortening; add
well beaten egg. Add dry ingredients
of sifted flour & salt to creamed
mixture alternately with milk.

Beat well & add sorghum & flavoring.

Bake in 350-degree oven until cake
springs back when pressed
with hand.

Rhubarb Pie (1)

2-Egg   3 tbs flour
1 C.   cup sugar

Sour cream cake

1. Butter Yellow CAKE mix
2/3 cup Wesson oil
½ cup Sugar
4 eggs

1 cup nuts

1 cup Sour cream

pour half of mixture in Baking pan
Sprinkel Sugar + cinnamon mixture
add remaning Batter Bake 350 for 1 hour

6 TSP. Brown Sugar
6 TSP Cinnamon

5 Cups sugar
1 cup Corn syrup
1 Cup water
2 eggs white
boil sugar syrup water until
it forms a hard Ball when dropped in
water pour over beaten egg whites
add cup nuts Cherries 1 ½ Vanilla

2. tabl½ egg... beaten
1. tab 2 cups Rhubarb Cut in...
½ teas 1 rei...

MISSISSIPPI Mud Cake

2 Cups Sugar
1 Cup wesson oil
⅓ Cup Cocoa
1½ Cups Flour
4 eggs
1 Cup pecans
2 teaspoons vanilla
¼ teaspoon salt

Cream Sugar eggs Beat well Stir in
flour, Cocoa & Salt to mixture add
remaining ingredients. Bake at 300°
for 40 to 45 min
Pour 1 Small pack of marshmellows
over cake, Brown lightly

Topping

1 Stick margarine
½ Cup Milk
1 Box Confectionary Sugar
1 Cup pecans
Spread on Hot Cake

Corn Relish

8 - cups corn
1 - cup Chopped onions
1 - cup Chopped green Sweet Pepper
1 - cup Chopped Red Pepper (Sweet)
4 - cups Chopped cabbage
2 - tablespoon mustard
1 - tablespoon mustard seed
1 - Tablespoon salt
1 - Tablespoon Turmic
1½ to 2 cups sugar
4 - cups vinegar

Boil corn 5 minutes - Cut from
cob. Mix all ingredients with 1-
cup water. Simmer 20 minutes,
Bring to a boil. Pack boiling
hot into jars & seal. Makes
about 8 pints.

James D. Gadberry
Route 5
Russell Springs, Kentucky 42642

Sorghum Cake

1 egg well beaten

1½ cup sorghum

1 stick butter or other shortening

½ cup milk or buttermilk

1 tsp soda

1 tsp baking powder

2½ cups flour
1 tsp flavoring

Pear Honey

5 lb. sugar

4 lb. pears grind.
1 can pineapple
cup.

Cook 40 Min.

Cook pears + pin.
together + grind
+ surejell foam
up + jelly

Cover top crust or lattice & bake in
hot oven (425) 10 minutes: reduce
temperature (350) and bake 35 minutes
longer. makes 1. 9 inch pie

Lemon Pie

1 - cup flour
1½ - cups sugar
4 - egg yolks
The juice from 1 lemon
Milk

Mix sugar & flour — add milk & butter
Cook until forms hard boil — Beat —

Add Marshmellow & beat until smooth

Molasses Cake

3/4 cup shortening
1/2 cup brown sugar
3 eggs
3/4 cup molasses
2 cups + 2 tbs. All purpose flour
1½ tsp. baking powder
3/4 tsp. soda
3/4 tsp. salt
1½ tsp. cinnamon
1½ tsp. ginger
3/4 cup boiling water

Jam Cake

2 cups Brown Sugar
2 cups Butter milk
1 cup rasins
3½ cups flour flour
2 teaspoons of soda
1 Tablespoon cocoa
1 cup Butter
one cup jam
1 cup chopped nuts
3 eggs - seperated
1 teaspoon cinnamon
1 teaspoon cloves

Topping

2 cups brown sugar
2 teaspoons flour
½ cup milk
2 Tablespoons butter
2 Tablespoons of Marshmallow Whip

Cream shortening, sugar & vanilla – add one egg at a time – beat well after each. Make a mixture of cocoa & food coloring in a small dish – add to mixture. Sift flour & salt – add flour & buttermilk alternately – start with flour & end with flour. Combine <u>soda</u> & <u>vinegar</u> & <u>as a last</u> to batter & beat well. Bake in sheet pan or 3 greased & floured 9" cake pans at 350° for 30 min.

DISH

PREPARATION TIME
NUMBER OF SERVINGS
SOURCE OF RECIPE

Red Velvet Cake

1 c. margarine
2 eggs
1 t. vanilla
1 t. salt
1 t. soda
1 T. vinegar
1½ c. sugar
2 oz. red food coloring
1 T. cocoa

1 c. buttermilk
2½ c. flour

Cucumber Pickles (2)

Slice cucumbers cross ways. put them in
a mixture of lime & water in
enameled or pottery container let
stand overnight. Remove from lime-
water, wash cucumbers through
three changes of fresh, cold water
Mix vinegar, sugar, & salt & place
drained cucumber slices in mixture

Cucumber Pickles   (1)

8 lbs. cucumbers
2 cups household lime
2 gal. water
2 pts. vinegar
9 cups sugar
2 tablespoons salt

Cucumber Pickles (2)

Slice cucumbers cross ways. put them in
a mixture of lime & water in
enameled or pottery container let
stand overnight. Remove from lime -
water, wash cucumbers through
three changes of fresh cold water
Mix. vinegar, sugar, & salt & place
drained cucumber slices in mixture

Cucumbers Pickles (1)

8 lbs. cucumbers
2 cups household lime
2 gal. water
2 pts. vinegar
9 cups sugar
2 tablespoons salt

Butter Milk Pie

3 eggs
2 cups sugar
1 stick margarine
½ cup butter milk
2 Tablespoons flour
1 teaspoon vanilla
Bake in unbaked pie shell
350 degree

Chicken Salad

2 cups chicken, diced
2 cups celery, chopped (onions & etc.)
2 hard-boiled eggs, sliced
salt & pepper
salad dressing

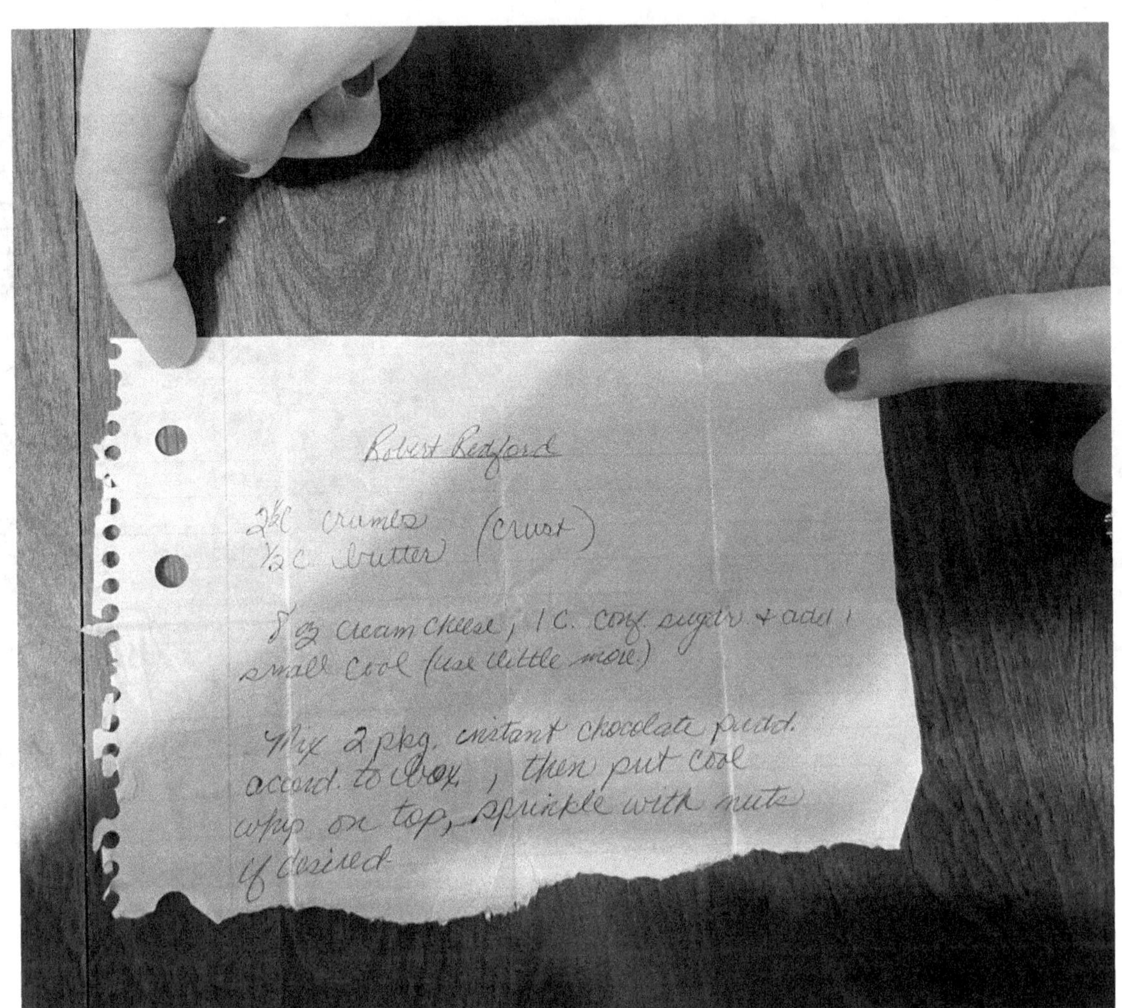

Robert Redford

2½C crumbs (crust)
½ C butter

8 oz cream cheese, 1 C. conf. sugar & add 1
small cool (use little more)

Mix 2 pkg. instant chocolate pudd.
accord. to box, then put cool
whip on top, sprinkle with nuts
if desired.

<u>Robert Redford</u>

2½C crumbs (crust)
½ C butter

8 oz cream cheese, 1 C. conf. sugar + add 1
small Cool (use a little more.)

Mix 2 pkg. instant chocolate pudd.
accord. to box, then put cool
whip on top, sprinkle with nuts
if desired.

Pecan Pie

1 - cup Brown Sugar
½ cup White Sugar
1 tables flour
2 eggs
2 tables milk
1 tsp Vanilla
½ cup Butter melted
1 - cup Pecan

Mix Sugar & flour and add
beaten eggs, milk, vanilla & butter
beat until smooth, fold in
pecans & put in pie crust.
Bake at 325 for one hour.

This is Day 5

Amish Friendship Cake

Do not refrigerate starter.
Do not use metal spoon to stir.
Day 1 - Do nothing
Day 2-4 - stir
Day 5 - add 1 cup flour, 1 cup milk, + 1 cup sugar. Stir.
Day 6-9 - Stir
Day 10 - add 1 cup flour, 1 cup sugar, + 1 cup milk.
Pour into 3 separate containers (1 cup each) give to 2
friends with these instructions. Keep one for yourself.

To the remaining batter Add: $\frac{2}{3}$ cup oil, 2 cups flour.
1 cup sugar
1$\frac{1}{4}$ tsp baking powder
1$\frac{1}{2}$ tsp. cinnamon
1 tsp. soda. 2 tsp. vanilla
3 eggs
1 large box Vanilla instant pudding.
1 cup nuts.
Add $\frac{3}{4}$ cup milk if mixture is too thick. Pour into
3 loaf pans or 1 bundt pan.
    Bake 40-45 minutes at 350°
Cool 10 min. before removing from pan.

Brown Sugar pie

2 cups brown Sugar
½ cups White Sugar
⅔ cups Flour
4 Eggs yellows
3 tablespoons Butter
2½ cups Milk
teaspoons Vanilena

Zucchini Cake

2 cups zucchini (shredded)
Add 3 eggs (well beaten)
2 - cups sugar
1 - cup veg. oil
1 - teaspoon vanilla
3 - cups flour
3 - teaspoon cinnamon
½ - cup nuts
Mix ingredients together. Bake at 350

Glaze

2 - cups confictioner sugar
2 - tablespoon water
2 - tablespoon syrup
2 - tablespoon soft butter
1 - teaspoon vanilla
Mix together and spread over warm
cake.

Footnote:-
For zucchini bread use 4 tsp. baking powder
Bake in 2 well greased and floured loaf pans
for 45 minutes or longer at 325 degrees

Zucchini Cake

2 cups zucchini (shredded)
Add 3 eggs (well beaten)
2 - cups sugar
1 - cup veg. oil
1 - teaspoon vanilla
3 - cups flour
3 - teaspoon cinnamon
½ - cup nuts
Mix ingredients together. Bake at 350

Glaze

2 - Cups Confectioner sugar
2 - tablespoon Water
2 - tablespoon syrup
2 - tablespoon soft butter
1 - teaspoon vanilla
Mix together and spread over warm cake.

Footnote:
For zucchini bread use 4 tsp. baking powder
Bake in 2 well greased and floured loaf pans
for 45 minutes or longer at 325 degrees

Cresco Icing

1 - box powdered sugar
cup full of butter Cake
flavoring
1 - teaspoon Vanilla
1/3 - cup milk
1 - cup Cresco

Mix all ingredients
together
beat well

Dill Pickles

Scrub 25-30 4-inch cucumbers. Pack into hot sterilized quart jars. To each jar add 2 tsp. Durkees dill seed, 1 lump of Durkees alum (size of pea), & 1 tsp. Durkees mustard seed. Fill jars with hot brine, allowing 1 tablesp. coarse salt, 1 C. vinegar & 1½ C. water for each quart jar. Seal jars. Let stand 5 to 7 days before serving.

Red Velvet Cake

1 Box White Cake Mix
1 Box Instant Vanilla Pudding Mix
2 oz red food coloring
2 eggs
3/4 cup oil
1 cup water
1/4 teaspoon Vanilla
1/4 teaspoon Almond
1 tablespoon Chocolate (cocoa) mixed in
a little water.
Bake at 350° for 30 or 35 min.

Butter Cream Frosting

1 lb. Confectionary Sugar

1/2 Stick Butter

3 tablespoons milk

1 teaspoon Vanilla cake
flavoring

mix milk one spoon
full at a time, Thicken
with Confectionary Sugar
or thin down with more
milk,

Chocolate Icing

2 - cups Confectioners sugar
6 - tablespoons butter
4 - tablespoons cocoa
1 - teaspoon vanilla — 3 - tablespoons strong coffee
Sift together sugar + cocoa + cream
into butter using necessary amount
of coffee and vanilla to obtain the
desired amount.

Chocolate Icing

2 - cups Confectioners sugar
6 - tablespoons butter
4 - tablespoons cacoa
1 - teaspoon vanilla — 3 - tablespoons strong coffee
Sift together sugar & cacoa & Cream
into butter using necessary amount
of coffee and vanilla to obtain the
desired amount.

Cinnamon Bread

2 cups flour
1½ tsp. cinnamon
2 eggs, beaten
2 cups sugar
1 cup milk

Topping:
½ cup sugar
1½ tsp. cinnamon
2 tsp. butter or margarine (melted)

Bake at 375°. Add your flour & cinnamon alternately with cup of milk.

"Chicken & Noodles Crock Pot"

2 - Cans of Cream of Chicken soup
2 - Cans Chicken broth (15 oz each)
1 - stick butter or margarine
1 lb. - chicken breast
1 - package frozen egg noodles (24 oz)

In crock pot put chicken on bottom.
Pour chicken broth + soup on top.
Top with stick of butter.
Put the crockpot on low for 6-7 hours.
Take chicken out and shred, put
back in crock pot. Add the noodles
+ cook 2 more hours, stir every
30 minutes until done.

In a small saucepan, mix together all
ingredients except the vanilla + the extra
2 Tablespoons of butter, Heat over medium heat
and bring to a boil, Stirring frequently
to prevent burning, let the mixture boil
for a good one minute (Make sure to
boil for a good solid minute)
Take off the fire and add vanilla the rest
of butter. Cool mixture occasionally giving
it a vigorous stir, until it is still warm
(but not hot) and his thickened enough to
spread, spread it over the cake moving
fairly quickly because it will set as it
cools, It will be a thin coating, not thick
layer, Let it set competety before Cutting
the cake.

"Butterscotch Cake"

2 - Cups Brown sugar
½ - C. Butter
1 - teaspoon vanilla
2 - eggs
2 - Cups flour
1 - teaspoon Soda
1 - teaspoon Baking Powder
½ - teaspoon salt
1 - cup Buttermilk

Preheat oven to 350 degress, grease & flour two
9" pans or 6" inch (3)
Cream the butter and sugar with electric mixer
on medium until fluffy, add vanilla, then add
eggs one at a time, beating on low just until they
are mixed in.
In a seperate bowl, sift together the flour,
baking soda, baking powder, & salt, Starting with
flour mixture, add the flour and the buttermilk
(alternating one then the other) into the sugar
egg mixture on low speed. When everything is
mixed in, scrape down the bowl by hand
Pour batter into the pans and bake for 25-30
minutes, until toothpick inserted in the
middle comes out clean. Cool before frosting

Caramel Frosting

1½ - Cups brown sugar
1 - tablespoon flour
¼ - cup butter (plus 2 tablespoon for later)
¼ - cup milk
¼ teaspoon vanilla
1 teaspoon vanilla

Over →

"Glazed Baby Carrots"

1 lb. fresh, frozen or canned whole ~~baby~~ Baby Carrots
2 tablespoon butter or margarine
¼ cup packed brown sugar
Cook carrots in a small amount of Water until tender. Drain. ~~In~~ a saucepan, combine butter and brown sugar, heat until sugar dissolves. Add carrots toss to coat. Heat through. (4 servings)

Butterscotch Pie

1 C brown Sugar
3 tb shortening (Butter)
4 tb cream
  Cook this mixture until thick
and brown. The browner it is
cooked, the more butterscotch taste
it has. To this add
  1 C milk   1 egg yolk
  6 level tb flour
Mix these ingredients well   (over)

and then with the fruit
mixture stirring constantly,
cook until thick & pour into
baked pie crust

"Quick Coconut Cream Pie"

1 - package (5.1 oz) instant Vanilla pudding
1½ - cups Cold Milk
1 - Carton (8oz) frozen Whipped topping (thawed, divided)
1 - pastry shell, baked or graham Cracker Crust.
In a mixing bowl, beat pudding + milk on low speed for 2 minutes. Fold in half of the whipped topping + ½ to ¾ cup of Coconut. Pour into Crust. Spread with remaining whipped topping, Sprinkle with remaining Coconut. Chill (6 to 8 servings)

"Butterscotch Cake"

2 – Cups Brown sugar
1/2 – C. Butter
1 – teaspoon vanilla
2 – eggs
2 – cups flour
1 – teaspoon Soda
1 – teaspoon Baking Powder
1/2 – teaspoon salt
1 – cup Buttermilk

Preheat oven to 350 degrees, grease & flour two
9" pans or 6 "inch (3)
Cream the butter and sugar with electric mixer
on medium until fluffy, add vanilla, then add
eggs one at a time, beating on low just until they
are mixed in.
In a seperate bowl, sift together the flour,
baking soda, baking powder, & salt, Starting with
flour mixture, add the flour and the buttermilk
(alternating one then the other) into the sugar
egg mixture on low speed, When everything is
mixed in, scrape down the bowl by hand
Pour batter into the pans and bake for 25 – 30
minutes, until toothpick inserted in the
middle comes out clean. Cool before frosting

Caramel Frosting

1 1/2 – Cups brown sugar
1 – tablespoon flour
1/4 – Cup butter (plus 2 tablespoon for later)
1/4 – Cup milk
1 teaspoon vanilla

over →

In a small saucepan, mix together all ingredients except the vanilla + the extra 2 Tablespoons of butter. Heat over medium heat and bring to a boil, stirring frequently to prevent burning. Let the mixture boil for a good one minute (Make sure to boil for a good solid minute)

Take off the fire and add vanilla the rest of butter. Cool mixture occasionally giving it a vigorous stir, until it is still warm (but not hot) and his thickened enough to spread. Spread it over the cake, moving fairly quickly because it will set as it cools. It will be a thin coating, not thick layer. Let it set competely before cutting the cake.

"Glazed Baby Carrots"
1 lb. fresh, frozen or canned whole Baby ~~Baby~~ Carrots
2-tablespoon butter or margarine
¼-cup packed brown sugar
Cook carrots in a small amount of Water
until tender. Drain. ~~In~~ a saucepan, Combine
butter and brown sugar, heat until sugar
dissolves. add carrots toss to coat.
Heat through. (4 servings)

and stir until the fruit
and these stirring constantly.
Cook until thick & pour into
baked pie crust

Butterscotch Pie

1 C brown Sugar
3 tb shortening (Butter)
4 tb cream
Cook this mixture until thick
and brown. The browner it is
cooked, the more butterscotch taste
it has. To this add
1 C. milk   1 - egg yolk
6 level tb flour
Mix these ingredients well (over)

"Quick Coconut Cream Pie"

1 - package (5.1 oz) instant Vanilla pudding
1½ - cups cold Milk
1 - carton (8 oz) frozen Whipped topping (thawed, divided)
1 - pastry shell, baked or graham Cracker Crust.

In a mixing bowl, beat pudding + Milk on low speed for 2 minutes. Fold in half of the whipped topping + ½ to ¾ cup of Coconut. Pour into Crust. Spread with remaining whipped topping, Sprinkle with remaining Coconut. Chill (6 to 8 servings)

Boy

Chocolate Cake Mix

8 oz Cream Cheese
1 stick butter or margarine
Cream together
add
3 cups powdered Sugar
add one cup at a time
+ Mix Well
Then add 8 oz ~~cup~~ bowl
of Cool Whip
Mix well
put between layers
of cake.

No Bake Praline Cookies

Sugar 1 ½ cup
Brown sugar 1 cup
Syrup ½ cup
Coconut 2 cups
Butter ½ cup
Pecans 2 - cups
Milk ½ cup Pet milk
Vanilla 1 teaspoon
Salt ½

↙ Bring to boil the ↙
sugars, syrup, butter and
milk

Take off stove add Vanilla,
Coconut, & Pecans, mix
together then drop by
tablespoon on wax paper
Let set.

"Royal Raspberry Cake"

2 - c. all purpose flour
1/2 - teaspoon Salt
1. tlB - Baking Powder
1/3 - Cup Margarine (Room Temp)
1 - C - Sugar

1 egg (room Temperature)
1 - C. Milk
1 - teaspoon Vanilla
3 1/2 C - fresh or frozen berries (unsweetened)

Stir together first three ingredients in a bowl with Wire Whisk, set aside. Cream softened Butter with Mixer. Add sugar gradually, beating Well after each addition, until mixture is fluffy & light. Stir in egg, beat 1 minute. Combine Milk + Vanilla, add

OVER →

"Sweet Potato Casserole"

3 - cups mashed Sweet Potatoes
1 - cup sugar
½ - cup butter
2 - eggs
1 - teaspoon vanilla
⅓ - cup evaporated Milk
½ - teaspoon cinnamon

"Topping"

Corn Casserole
1 can cream corn
1 can whole corn (drained)
2 eggs
1/4 cup sugar
1/2 cup sour cream
1/2 cup oil
1 box Jiffy cornbread mix
    (8 1/2 oz)

Mix together and bake
at 350° for 1 hour.

"Homemade Payday Candy Bars"

3 cups salted Peanuts
2 cup peanut butter chips
2 cups Mini Marshmallows
1 14oz can sweetened Condensed milk
3 tablespoon unsalted butter
1/2 - teaspoon Vanilla

Melt butter and peanut butter chips in large saucepan over medium heat until smooth then stir in Condensed milk, Vanilla extract + Marshmallows stirring until smooth + incorporated
Generously grease a 9X13 inch baking dish with butter or non stick spray or line with parchment paper, then spread half of peanuts across baking dish
Pour Condensed milk mixture over peanuts then sprinkle rest of peanuts on top

"Hawaiian Cinnamon Rolls"

A package of Hawaiian Buns (slice into)
2 sticks butter
Cinnamon + sugar
Spread over buns put together then roll
Out, more sugar + cinnamon (butter first)
Roll up slice + put into muffin pan.
Bake at 350° for 20 minutes.
Ice and enjoy make 1 dozen

"Heavenly Cherry Angel Food Trifle"

5 cups - Angel food cake cubes
8. oz - frozen whipped topping (Cool Whip)   may need larger Cool Whip
1/2 - cup toasted Chopped Nuts.
1 can - (21. oz) Cherry Pie Filling or topping.
Place cake cubes in large bowl. Mix Cool Whip + Nuts together, then mix with cake cubes. Layer with Cherry pie filling ending with Cherry Pie filling. 8-10 serving

"Slow Cooked Sage Dressing"

14 to 15 cups day-old bread cubes (9 cups cornbread

1½ - cups chopped onion

1½ - teaspoon rubbed sage

1 - teaspoon salt

½ - teaspoon pepper

1¼ cups butter or Margarine (melted) (or broth)

Combine bread, ~~celery~~, onion, sage, salt & pepper. Mix well. Add butter or broth & toss. Spoon into 5 qt slow Cooker. Cover & cook on low for 4-5 hours stirring once. (12 Servings)

"Coconut Cake"

1 - White Cake Mix
Egg whites - follow direction on box. *don['t] add wa[ter]*
1 - Can coconut milk
Mix & bake in 9x13 pan at 350° 25 to [.] m[in]

Frosting
1 - 8 oz bowl of Cool Whip
1 - tablespoon powdered sugar
Mix spread on cooled cakes.
Sprinkle with coconut

"Chocolate Cherry Cake"

1 - pk. (18.25 oz) fudge cake Mix

1 - can (21 oz) cherry pie filling

2 - eggs (beaten)

1 - tsp. almond extract

In mixing bowl, stir together all cake ingredients
Pour into a greased 13 x 9 x 2 in cake pan. Bake a[t]
350° for 30 Minutes or until cake test done.

"Strawberries in the Snow"

8 oz Cream Cheese
1. cup sugar ⎤ Blend
~~1/2 cup milk~~ ⎦ together

1/2 - cup milk ⎤ Blend
16 - oz Cool Whip ⎦ Together then mix with sugar + cheese

1 - large Angel Food cake
2 - pkg. Strawberry glaze
2 - boxes of strawberries
Break the angel food cake in bite size Chunks, layer
out

"Strawberry Cotton Candy Salad"

1 – Can sweeten Condensed milk
2 – Cups Crushed Pineapple (well drained)
1 – cup strawberry pie filling
12 OZ – tub Cool Whip
8 – large strawberries (halved)
3/4 – cup pecans (Chopped) (optional)
Fold all together and top with strawberries. Chill serve + enjoy

"Boston Poke Cake"

1 – box yellow cake mix
2 – boxes of instant vanilla Pudding mix
4 – Cups milk
1 – container of chocolate frosting

Prepare cake mix in 13×9 according to box directions, Bake at 350° for 30 minutes. Combine milk + pudding mix + Whisk until blended, Poke holes in cake Pour pudding over cake making sure it gets down into the holes. (Refrigate)

"Coca Cola Pork Loin"

1/4 - cup soy sauce
1 - cup coca Cola
1/2 - cup dark brown sugar
2 - Tb. Dijon mustard.
Put on pork loin and cook

"Coca Cola Pork Loin"

1/4 - Cup soy sauce
1 - Cup coca Cola
1/2 - Cup dark brown sugar
2 - Tb. Dijon mustard.
Put on pork loin and cook

Texas Roadhouse Butter

Copycat recipe

2 - sticks butter
1 - cup powdered sugar
1 - cup Honey
2 - teaspoon cinnamon
Mix all together until its the
~~consis~~ consistency you want

"Corn Candy Fudge"

Vanilla Chips
1 Can sweeten Condensed milk
2 tsp. Vanilla
Corn Candy

Melt chips stir in condensed milk
add vanilla stir in corn candy.
Put in pan and decorate with corn
candy. Let set and cut into squares

"Crescent Pie Bites

1 - (21 oz) can pie filling
2 - tubes Crescent Rolls
1 - cup powdered sugar
2 - tablespoons milk

Preheat oven 375 degrees
Spray two muffins tin with cooking spray
Open Crescent roll cans & lay out the crescent roll
dough flat.
Separate into individual sections and lay each
piece in the muffin tins, widest section
on bottom.
Put pie filling section on bottom
About 1 - 2 tablespoons per crescent, gather the edges of
the dough and fold around filling. Bake 12 to 15 minutes
                    Glaze

Mix powdered sugar and milk together until
smooth drizzle over each bite

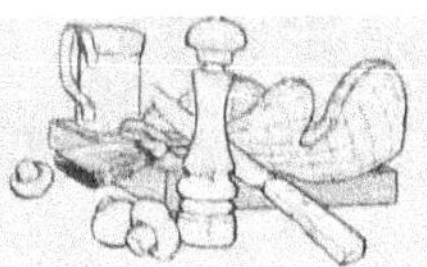
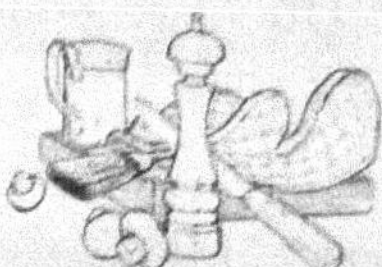

Recipe # _______________

Recipes from the kitchen of:

Betty Popplewell

Abbreviations to Use:

tsp. - teaspoons
tbsp. - tablespoons
C. - cup

pt. - pint
qt. - quart
lb. - pound

oz. - ounce
lg. - large
sm. - small

Category: _______________

Name Of Recipe: _Spam Meat Loaf_

INGREDIENTS

2-cans Spam (Shredded)
2-Eggs
1-onion (chopped)
1-10½ oz Can Tomato Puree
Cracker Crumbs (about 4 cups)
or you may need more Crumbs

DIRECTIONS

Shred Spam in Mixing bowl. (I use
my slaw shredder)
Add Cracker Crumbs, egg's, onion and
Tomato puree. Mix well. Line loaf
pan with reynolds wrap, put mixture
in loaf pan. Bake 1 Hour.
Bake about 30 minutes on 425°
Checking to see if it's getting to
brown, when you think its not
all the way through turn down
to 300° degree's + cook the
remaining hour.

"Sweet Baby Ray's Crockpot Chicken"

4 to 6 - Chicken breast
1 - bottle Sweet Baby Ray's sauce
1/4 - C. vinegar
1 - teaspoon red pepper flakes
1 - C. brown sugar
1/4 - teaspoon garlic powder

Mix everything together (except chicken)
Place chicken in crockpot (frozen is okay)
Pour sauce mixture over chicken.
Cook on low for 4 to 6 hours.

"Mandaran Orange Salad"

1 - box orange jello
1 - box instant vanilla pudding
1 - cup boiling water
½ - cup cold water
1 - Cool Whip (8 oz)
1 - can mandarin oranges drained (14 oz)
1 - cup mini Marshmallows

In a large bowl combine jello and boiling water whisk until jello is dissolved. Add cold water & allow to chill 15 minutes in frig. Slowly whisk in vanilla pudding mix until smooth and chill for another 15-20 minutes or until it becomes slightly thickened. Fold in Cool Whip, oranges & marshmallows

"Pumkin Bread"
1- box spice cake mix
1- Can (15 oz) pumkin
Mix & bake 350°

"Butter Pecan Cake"

2 2/3 - C. Chopped Nuts
1 1/4 - C. butter, softened. (diveded)
2 - C. sugar
4 - eggs
2 - tsp. vanilla
3 - Cups all purpose Flour
2 - tsp. baking powder
1/2 - tsp. salt
1 - C. milk
Place pecans + 1/4 Cup butter in a baking dish
over

"Old Fashion Banana Pudding"

2-cups sugar
4-egg yolks
enough flour to thicken
3 or 4 cups milk
mix and cook on stovetop or mironave

Norma Smith
Recipe

"Peach Dumplings"

2 - Whole large peaches
2 - 8 oz cans Cresent Rolls
2 - stick butter
1½ - C. sugar
1 - teaspoon vanilla
Cinnamon (to taste)
1½ - cups orange juice

Peel and pit peaches, Cut both peaches into 8 slices, Roll each peach slice in crescent roll, place in a 9X13 buttered pan. Melt butter, then add sugar and barely stir. add vanilla, stir and pour mixture over peaches. Pour orange juice around edges of the pan, Sprinkle with cinnamon + bake at 350 degrees for 40 minutes. Serve with ice cream + spoon some of the sweet sauces from pan over the top.

"Carmel Sauce"

1 - Cup Brown Suga
1/2 - stick Butter
1/2 - Cup Half & Half
1 - tablespoon vanilla
Pinch of salt

Mix all ingredients in a medium saucepan over medium low heat. Cook while whisking gently for 5 to 7 minutes until thicker Turn off heat, Serve warm or Cold

If sauce is thin just continue cooking for a few more minutes.

"Fruit Salad"

1 - (8 oz) Whipped topping (Cool whip)
2½ - C. Cocoanut
1½ C. Walnuts
1 - 8 oz can fruit cocktail (drained)
1 - 8 oz can pineapple chunks (drained)
1 - 11 oz mandarin oranges (drained)
3 - cups minature marshmallows

Mix all together.

"Chocolate Frosting"

1 - stick of butter
3 - tablespoon cocoa
6 - " " of cream or milk
1 - teaspoon vanilla
3 3/4 - cups powdered sugar

In a saucepan, combine the butter, cocoa and milk. Heat until butter melts. Beat in remaining ingredients and spread on the cake while its still warm.

"Mounds Bars"

2 – Cups of melted chocolate
3 – Cup Coconut
1 – Cup sweetened Condensed milk

Melt Chocolate
Mix coconut + milk together
Roll into whatever shape you
want + dip in chocolate

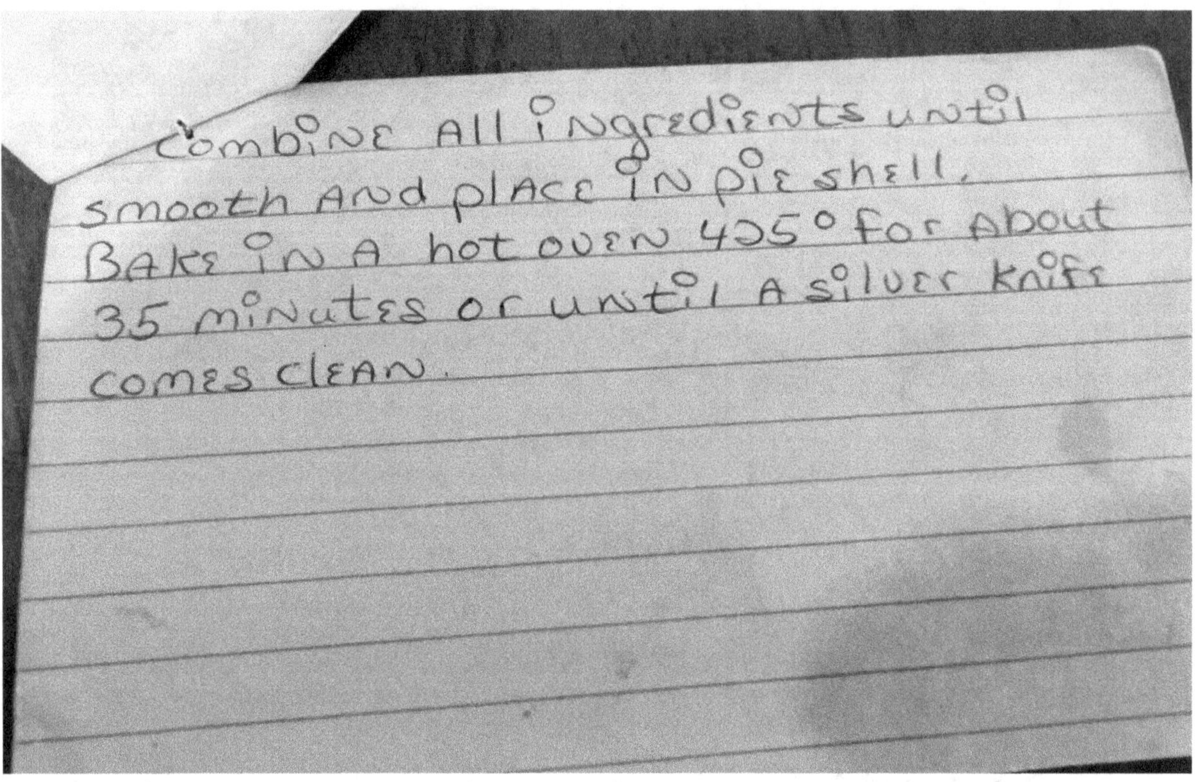
Combine all ingredients until
smooth and place in pie shell.
Bake in a hot oven 425° for about
35 minutes or until a silver knife
comes clean.

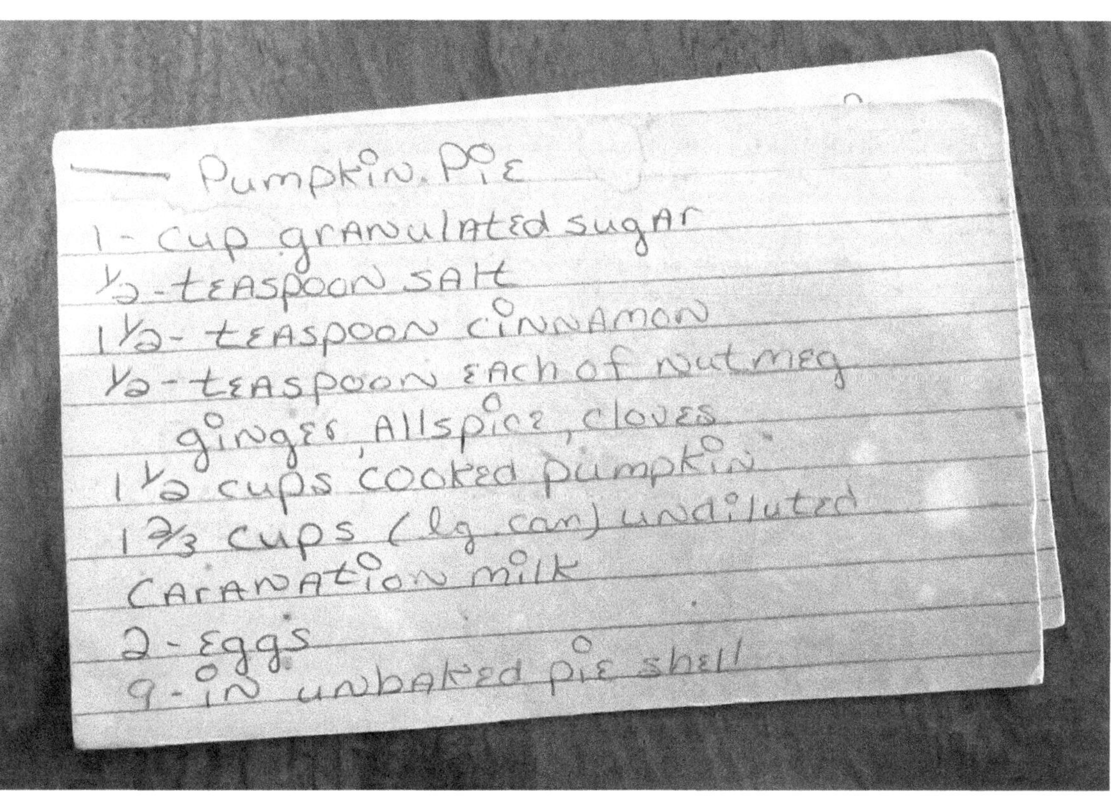

Pumpkin Pie
1 - cup granulated sugar
½ - teaspoon salt
1½ - teaspoon cinnamon
½ - teaspoon each of nutmeg
    ginger, Allspice, cloves
1½ cups cooked pumpkin
1⅔ cups (lg. can) undiluted
Carnation milk
2 - eggs
9 - in unbaked pie shell

Recipe: **Blueberry Dessert**
From: Velma
Makes: ___________________

1. Can Blueberry Pie Filling
1. large Box Vanilla instant Pudding
        (with 3 Cups Milk)
Graham Crackers
8 oz cool whip
    Whisk Vanilla Pudding + Milk until
thickened (couple Minutes) add Cool
whip. layer bottom pan with Graham
Crackers. Next layer Pudding Mixture.
keep layering. Top with Blueberry Pie Filling

STACK CAKE

1/2 cup shortening	6 cup flour
1 cup brown sugar	1/2 teaspoon soda
1 egg	1/2 teaspoon salt

1/2 cup molasses	1 teaspoon baking powder
1/2 cup buttermilk	1/2 teaspoon nutmeg

Cream shortening and sugar. Add egg and molasses. Beat well. Sift together dry ingredients. Add alternately to creamed mixture with buttermilk.

Divide dough in six parts. Roll and shape. Bake in 8" greased pan. Bake at 350° for 12 to 15 minutes.

Put together with dried apples mixture—cooked sieved apples flavored to taste with brown sugar and cinnamon. Ice cake with dried apple mixture.

"Old Fashion Muffins"

2 ¼ - cups flour
2 - eggs
½ cup shortening
1 - cup sugar
1 - cup milk
1 - tablespoon vanilla

Mix ~~dig~~ well (I don't use mixer)
+ put in muffin pan

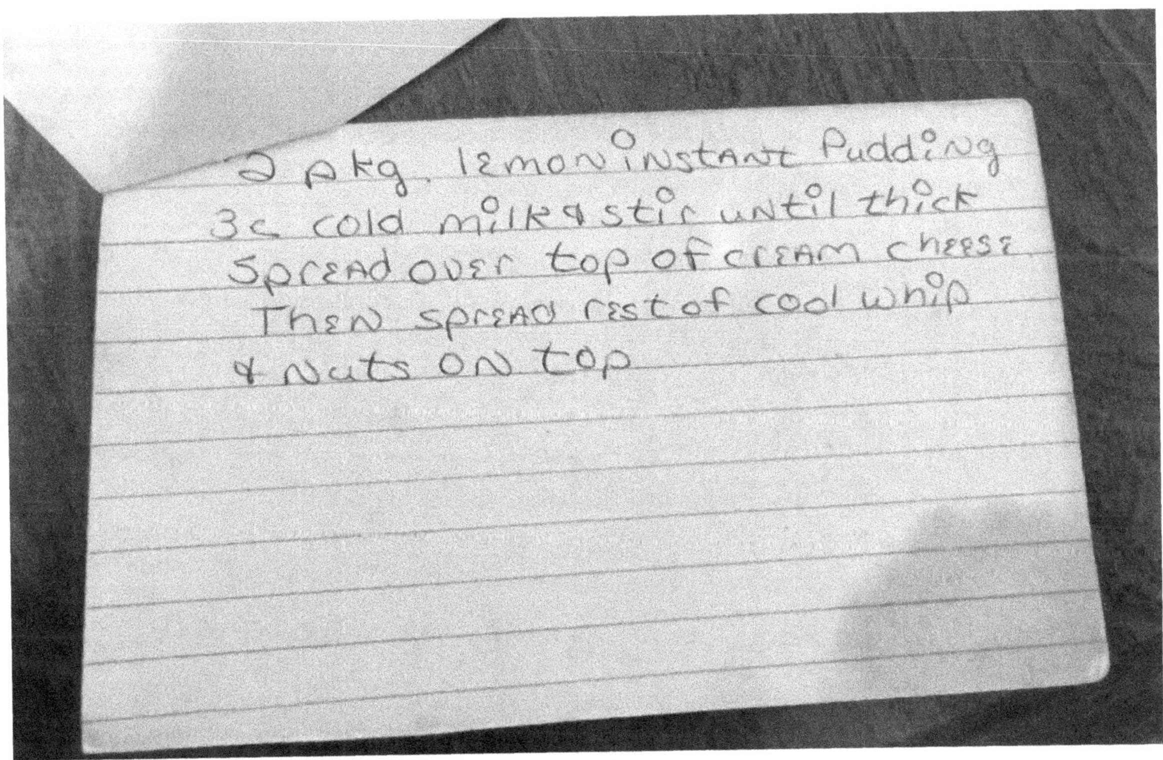

2 pkg. lemon instant Pudding
3c cold milk & stir until thick
spread over top of cream cheese
Then spread rest of cool whip
& nuts on top

Mother's Lemon Dessert

Mix 1 cup flour

1 stick melted butter

⅓ cup nuts   Mix this together

Put this out in bottom of pan &
bake 15 min. At 350°.

Mix the following.

8 oz cream cheese

1 c. cool whip

spread over crust layer

Then mix

Next Best Thing to Robert Redford

She uses Graham Cracker Crust for the
crust

1st Layer - Mix - 1 cup flour
1 stick butter or margarine
½ cup pecans
Press into 9×13" pan & bake 12 min. - Cool.

2nd Layer - Mix 1 pkg. instant chocolate pudding
according to box. put on 1st layer. Let cool

3rd Layer - Mix. 8 oz. cream cheese, 1 cup confectioners
sugar & ½ 1 small cool whip. Pour on 3rd layer.
Sprinkle with ½ cup pecans. Chill & serve

Brown Sugar Frosting (1.)

1 cup brown sugar (firmly packed)
⅓ cup water
¼ teaspoon cream of tarter
2 egg whites

Combine sugar water & cream of tarter, boil until syrup spins thread, beat egg whites until stiff, beat in hot syrup, & continue beating

Cornbread Dressing

1 cup chopped onion
4 cups chopped celery
1 cup shortening
1 tablespoon salt
½ teaspoon pepper
2 teaspoons poultry
  seasoning

7 cups bread cubes
9 cups cornbread crumbs
1½ to 2 cups broth,
  milk, or water
4 eggs, beaten

Cook onion and celery in shortening over low heat until onion is soft but not browned, stirring occasionally. Meanwhile, blend seasonings with bread cubes and cornbread crumbs. Add the onion and celery. Mix well. Gradually pour liquid and beaten eggs over the surface, stirring lightly. Add more seasonings as desired. Yield: stuffing for a 14- to 18-pound turkey.

"Crisco Icing"

1 - box powdered sugar
1 - cup crisco
Capful butter flavoring
Teaspoon vanilla
⅓ C - milk

Mix well together

"Cool Whip Frosting"

1 - 4 oz box instant pudding (dry any flavor)

1/4 - cup powdered sugar

1 - cup milk

1 - 8 oz package thawed Cool Whip

Add pudding mix, powdered sugar + milk to a mixing bowl. Mix on low speed until blended. Let mixture stand 3 minutes. Fold in Cool Whip. Frost + keep refrigerated.

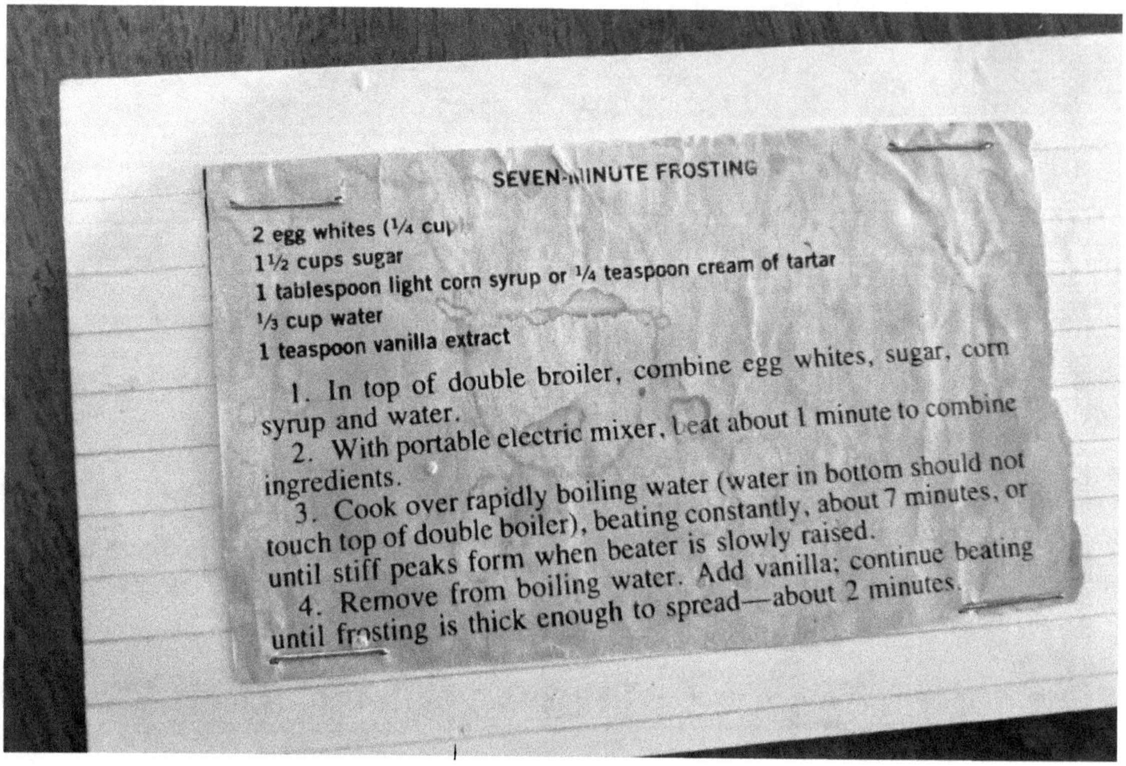

SEVEN-MINUTE FROSTING

2 egg whites (¼ cup)
1½ cups sugar
1 tablespoon light corn syrup or ¼ teaspoon cream of tartar
⅓ cup water
1 teaspoon vanilla extract

1. In top of double broiler, combine egg whites, sugar, corn syrup and water.
2. With portable electric mixer, beat about 1 minute to combine ingredients.
3. Cook over rapidly boiling water (water in bottom should not touch top of double boiler), beating constantly, about 7 minutes, or until stiff peaks form when beater is slowly raised.
4. Remove from boiling water. Add vanilla; continue beating until frosting is thick enough to spread—about 2 minutes.

~~Cat~~

Cat Head Biscuits

3½. C. self Rising Flour

¼ C. Oil

1¼ C. Buttermilk

¼ C. Butter

Pinch salt

Preheat oven 500 degrees

Using a mixing bowl add flour then milk pour oil over milk, Take a tablespoon and mix until well incorporated forming a ball, Pour dough onto a flat floured surface, sprinkle with flour. Now sprinkle flour lightly over dough, Take hands and press out to 1 in. thickness, Take a large biscuit cutter and cut out biscuits. Use excess dough by re-forming into a ball and onto a lightly greased baking sheet. Bake until lightly brown. Brush tops with butter if desired. Serve hot.

Pumpkin Pie →

Pumpkin Pie

1 — Can pumpkin (15 oz Can)
1 — Can Sweetened Milk (Condensed) (14 oz)
½ — tsp. Nutmeg
½ — tsp. Ginger
½ — teaspoon vanilla Cinnamon
1 — teaspoon salt
½ —

Pie Crust 9 inch

Preheat oven to 4 2 5 for 15 minutes
Reduce 350% cook/
35 or 40 minutes

- Prepare Lasagna Noodles as directed on the package.
  Pour Hot water off, and cover Lasagna with cold water.
  Set aside until noodles are needed.
- As noodles cook, saute the onion in the canola oil until
  onion is tender.   Remove from heat. Add the mushrooms,
  garlic powder, crushed red pepper, black pepper, and
  kidney beans. Stir well. Set aside.
- In a medium sized bowl, combine beaten eggs, Ricotta,
  Cottage, Parmasean, and Romano Cheeses, and about 8 ounces
  of the Mozzarella Cheese.   Set aside.
- Preheat oven to 350.
- Smear the inside of a 15" x 9" baking dish with non-stick spray.
- Spread 1/2 cup of Prego (right from the jar) in bottom of pan.
- Gently lift the Lasagna noodles one by one from the cold water.
  Hold them up a few seconds to drain, then lay them in the bottom
  of the pan, overlapping about half way.
- Spread half of the cheese mixture on top of the Lasagna noodles.
  Top the cheese mixture with half the onion mixture.
  Top the onion mixture with a generous amount of Prego.
  Layer the remaining ingredients in this order:
       Lasagna noodles, cheese mixture, onion mixture, Prego
  Sprinkle the rest of the Mozzarella cheese over the top,
  making sure to get all the way to the edges. Now sprinkle
  the top with Parsley Flakes.
- Spray a large sheet of foil with non-stick spray.
- Shape foil into a "tent", and place loosely over the Lasagna.
- Bake for one hour.
- Uncover, and bake until cheese on top is brown and bubbly.
- Remove from oven and let Lasagna stand about 15 minutes
  before serving. Slice and serve.

VEGETARIAN LASAGNA
Mary Susan Kerr

Ingredients:

1 lb. Lasagna Noodles
1 large Onion, sliced
1 4.5-oz. jar Green Giant Sliced Mushrooms, drained
1 16-oz. can Kidney Beans, well drained
1   tsp. Crushed Red Pepper
1/2 tsp. Coarse Grind Black Pepper
1/2 tsp. Italian Seasoning
1/4 tsp. garlic powder
2 eggs, well beaten
2 Tbs. Grated Parmasean Cheese
2 Tbs. Grated Romano Cheese
8-oz. Ricotta Cheese
8-oz. Large Curd Cottage Cheese
2 8-oz. pkg. Sargento 6-Cheese Italian Recipe Blend (gourmet shred)
2 12-oz. pkg. Kraft Finely Shredded Low-Moisture Part-Skim Mozzarella
2 large jars Prego Traditional Spaghetti Sauce
Parsley Flakes
Non-stick Spray

PEANUT BUTTER FUDGE

2 cups sugar

2/3 cup milk

Bring to boil and let form soft ball

when dropped into water. Take off

heat and beat in;

1 cup marshmallow cream

1 cup peanut butter

1 tsp. vanilla

Pour into buttered dish, cut when

cool.

Modine Vaught

EASY YEAST ROLLS

Joyce Stephens

1 egg
1 pkg. dry yeast
1/4 c. sugar
1 tsp. salt

1/3 c. shortening
1 c. milk
3 c. flour

Melt shortening and add milk. Cool to lukewarm. Add yeast.
Beat eggs and add with the sugar and salt to the milk mixture.
When the yeast is dissolved, add flour. Beat until well blended.
This will be a soft dough. Cover and refrigerate overnight or
several hours. Roll out on lightly floured board and shape or cut
out and dip lightly in butter. Place in a pan to let rise. When
double in size, bake at 400° for about 15 minutes or until brown.

BROCCOLI CORNBREAD

Joyce Stephens

10 ozs. chopped broccoli,
thawed and drained
1 c. chopped onion
1 small carton light sour cream

1 stick melted margarine
4 eggs
1 box Jiffy corn meal muffin mix

Beat eggs, then add all other ingredients with muffin mix last.
Mix. Bake 20 to 30 minutes in a large iron skillet sprayed with
Pam in a 400° oven. Goes well with soup.

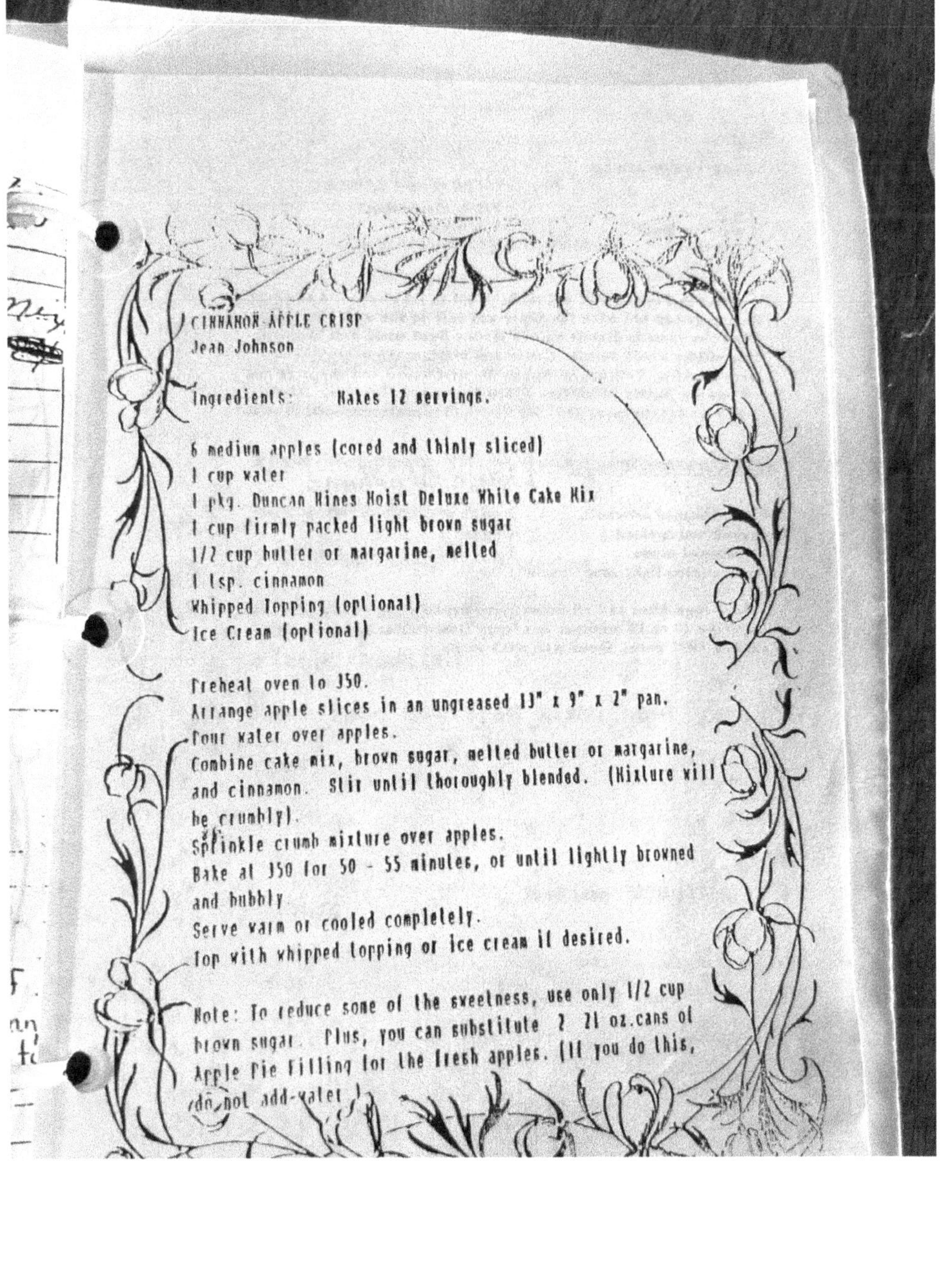

CINNAMON APPLE CRISP
Jean Johnson

Ingredients: Makes 12 servings.

6 medium apples (cored and thinly sliced)
1 cup water
1 pkg. Duncan Hines Moist Deluxe White Cake Mix
1 cup firmly packed light brown sugar
1/2 cup butter or margarine, melted
1 tsp. cinnamon
Whipped Topping (optional)
Ice Cream (optional)

Preheat oven to 350.
Arrange apple slices in an ungreased 13" x 9" x 2" pan.
Pour water over apples.
Combine cake mix, brown sugar, melted butter or margarine,
and cinnamon. Stir until thoroughly blended. (Mixture will
be crumbly).
Sprinkle crumb mixture over apples.
Bake at 350 for 50 - 55 minutes, or until lightly browned
and bubbly.
Serve warm or cooled completely.
Top with whipped topping or ice cream if desired.

Note: To reduce some of the sweetness, use only 1/2 cup
brown sugar. Plus, you can substitute 2 21 oz.cans of
Apple Pie Filling for the fresh apples. (If you do this,
do not add water.)

Mt. Dew Cake
Kim Johnson

1 Box Lemon Supreme Cake Mix
1 Box Lemon Instant Pudding
4 eggs
3/4 cup oil
10 z. Mt. Dew or 1 1/4 cup
Mix Well
Bake on 375   40 mins.

Cinnamon Bun Cake
1 Box Yellow Cake Mix
3/4 cup oil
4 eggs
1 cup Buttermilk
1 cup Brown sugar
1 table spoon cinnamon

mix 1st 4 ingredients together by hand. pour 1/2 of
mixture in 11 X 13 greased pan. mix brown sugar + cinn
together + sprinkle over batter. Add remaining batter to
pan. Then swirl with knife.
    Bake 40 minutes at 350°

Icing   2 cups confectioners sugar
        4 table spoon milk
        1 tsp vanilla
mix together + pour over hot cake.
Lawler Connie

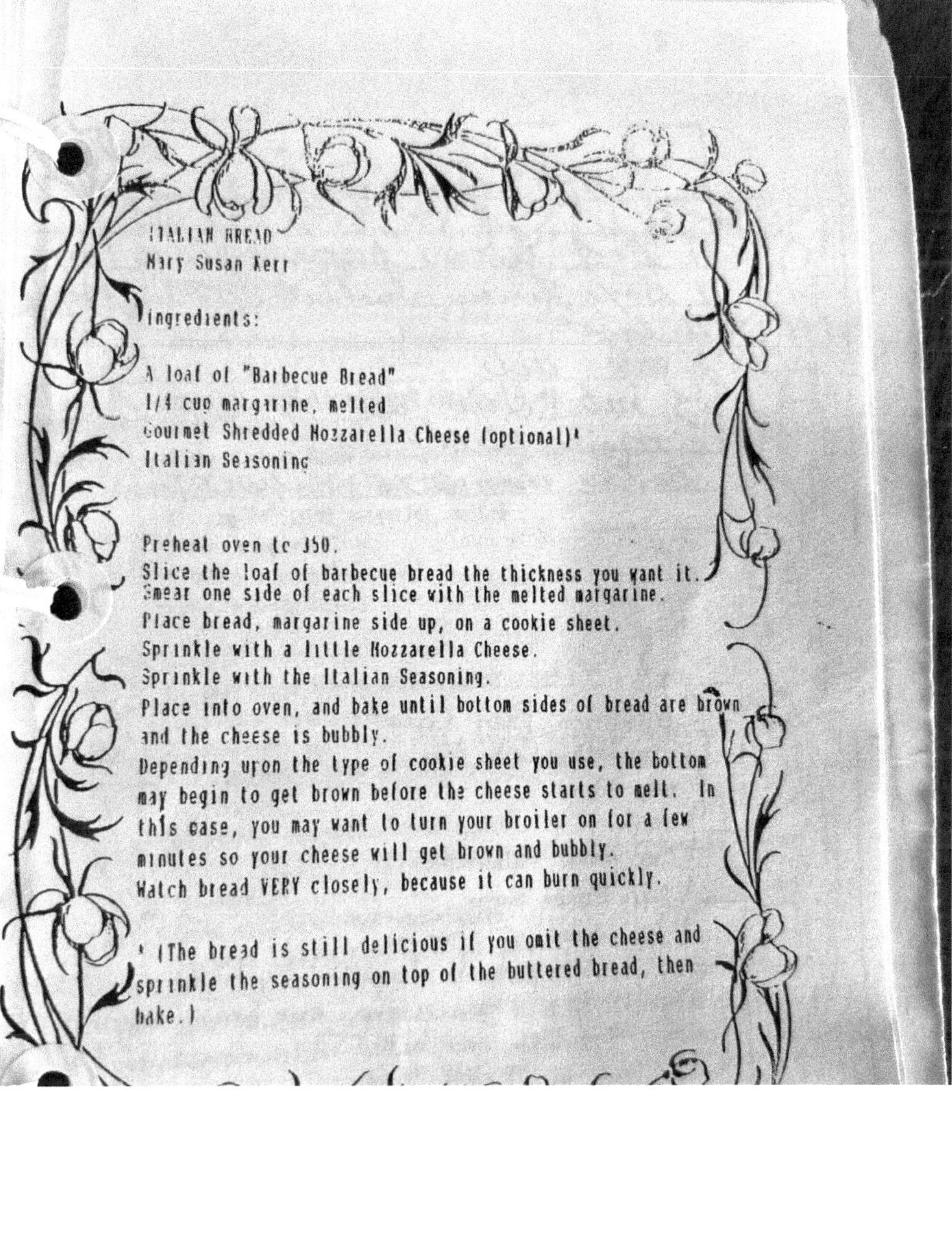

ITALIAN BREAD
Mary Susan Kerr

Ingredients:

A loaf of "Barbecue Bread"
1/4 cup margarine, melted
Gourmet Shredded Mozzarella Cheese (optional)*
Italian Seasoning

Preheat oven to 350.
Slice the loaf of barbecue bread the thickness you want it.
Smear one side of each slice with the melted margarine.
Place bread, margarine side up, on a cookie sheet.
Sprinkle with a little Mozzarella Cheese.
Sprinkle with the Italian Seasoning.
Place into oven, and bake until bottom sides of bread are brown
and the cheese is bubbly.
Depending upon the type of cookie sheet you use, the bottom
may begin to get brown before the cheese starts to melt. In
this case, you may want to turn your broiler on for a few
minutes so your cheese will get brown and bubbly.
Watch bread VERY closely, because it can burn quickly.

* (The bread is still delicious if you omit the cheese and
sprinkle the seasoning on top of the buttered bread, then
bake.)

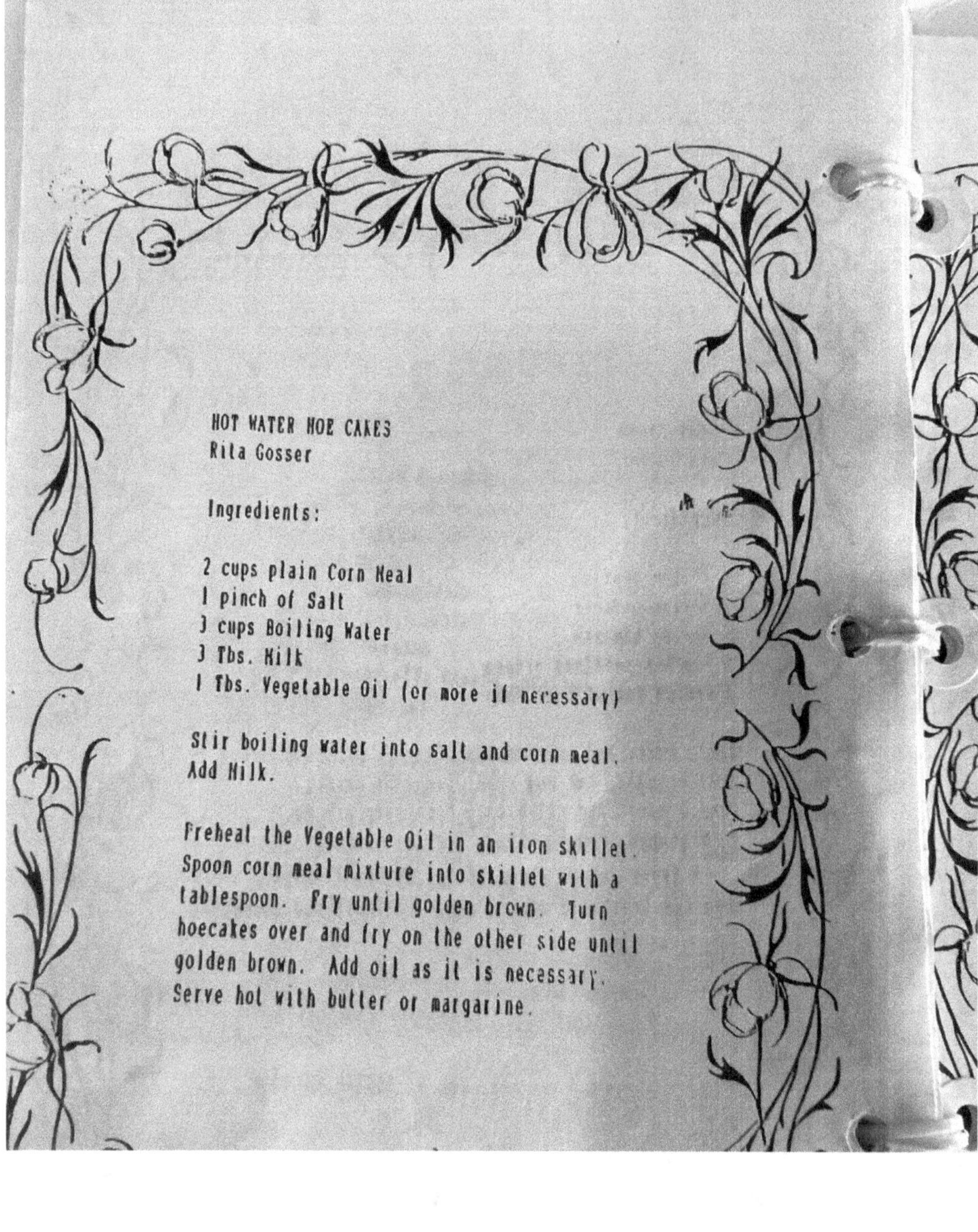

HOT WATER HOE CAKES
Rita Gosser

Ingredients:

2 cups plain Corn Meal
1 pinch of Salt
3 cups Boiling Water
3 Tbs. Milk
1 Tbs. Vegetable Oil (or more if necessary)

Stir boiling water into salt and corn meal.
Add Milk.

Preheat the Vegetable Oil in an iron skillet.
Spoon corn meal mixture into skillet with a
tablespoon. Fry until golden brown. Turn
hoecakes over and fry on the other side until
golden brown. Add oil as it is necessary.
Serve hot with butter or margarine.

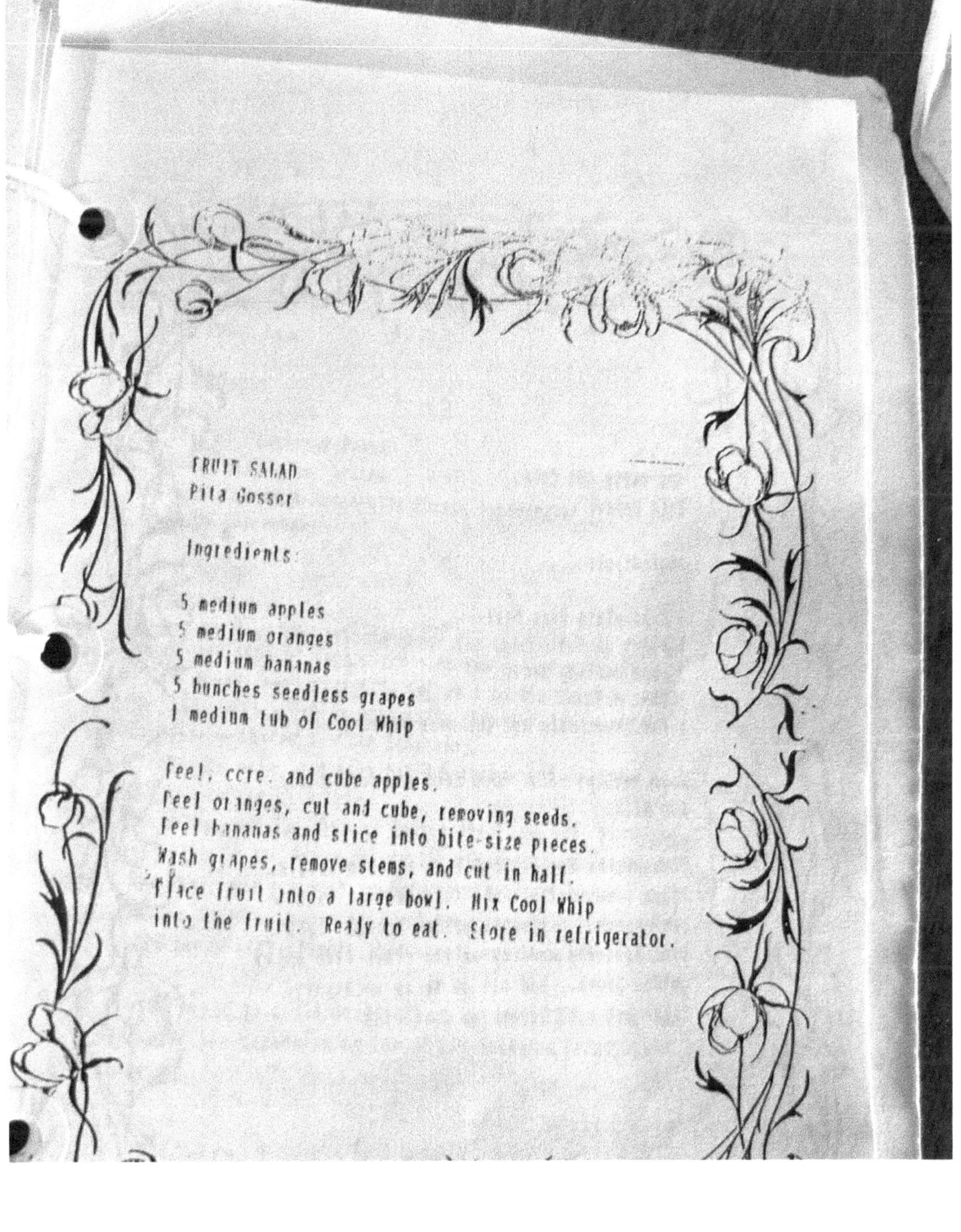

FRUIT SALAD
Pita Gosser

Ingredients:

5 medium apples
5 medium oranges
5 medium bananas
5 bunches seedless grapes
1 medium tub of Cool Whip

Peel, core, and cube apples.
Peel oranges, cut and cube, removing seeds.
Peel bananas and slice into bite-size pieces.
Wash grapes, remove stems, and cut in half.
Place fruit into a large bowl. Mix Cool Whip
into the fruit. Ready to eat. Store in refrigerator.

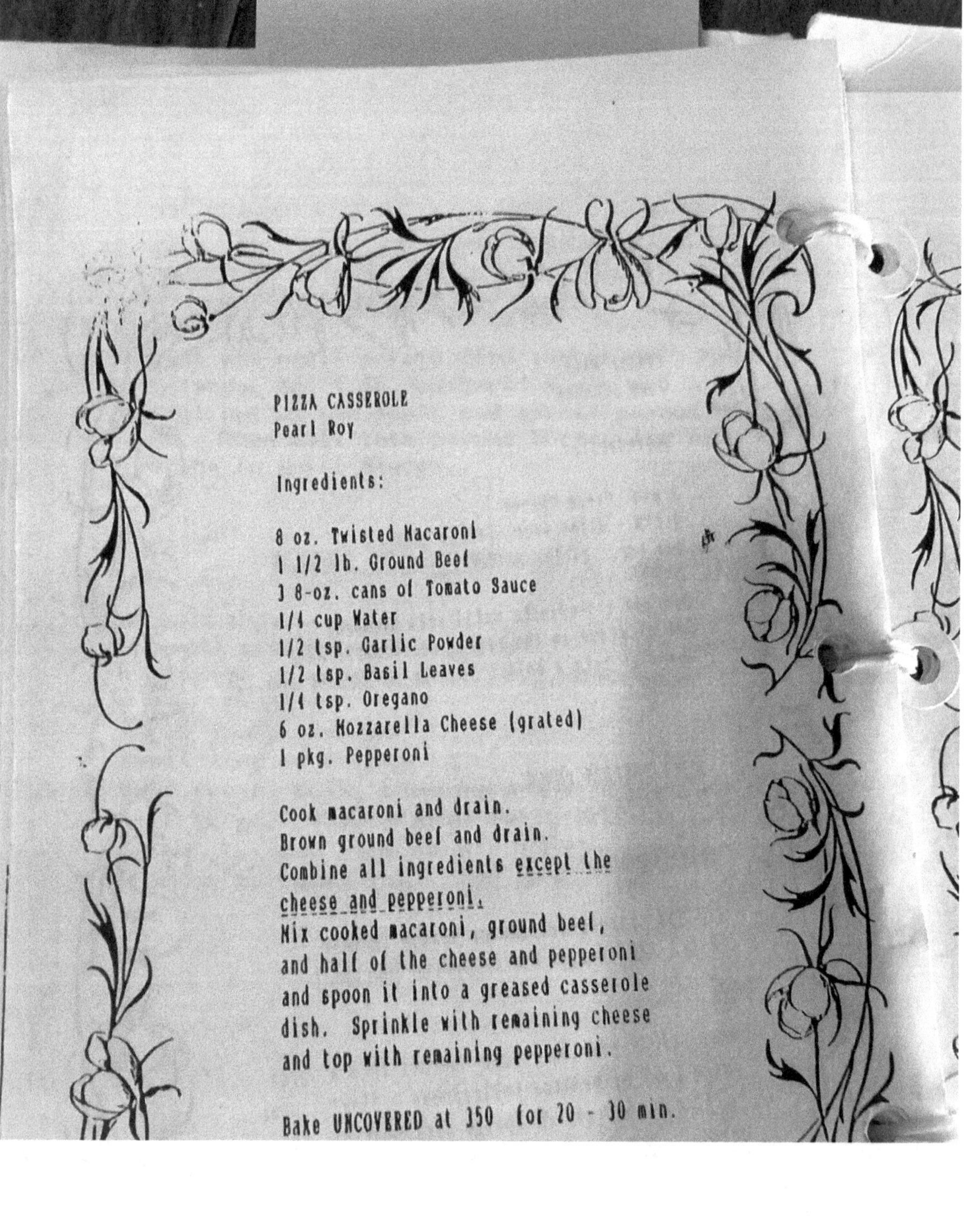

PIZZA CASSEROLE
Pearl Roy

Ingredients:

8 oz. Twisted Macaroni
1 1/2 lb. Ground Beef
3 8-oz. cans of Tomato Sauce
1/4 cup Water
1/2 tsp. Garlic Powder
1/2 tsp. Basil Leaves
1/4 tsp. Oregano
6 oz. Mozzarella Cheese (grated)
1 pkg. Pepperoni

Cook macaroni and drain.
Brown ground beef and drain.
Combine all ingredients except the
cheese and pepperoni.
Mix cooked macaroni, ground beef,
and half of the cheese and pepperoni
and spoon it into a greased casserole
dish. Sprinkle with remaining cheese
and top with remaining pepperoni.

Bake UNCOVERED at 350 for 20 - 30 min.

CHEESE BALL
Jean Johnson

Ingredients:

1 pkg. Cream Cheese
1 pkg. dried beef, finely chopped
1/4 tsp. garlic powder

Mix all ingredients until well blended.
Let it stand in the refrigerator until cold.
Shape it into a ball. Roll it in nuts if desired.

QUICK SHERBET PUNCH
Jean Johnson

Ingredients:

1/2 gal. pineapple lime or orange sherbet
10 1/2 gal. Ginger Ale or Sprite (chilled)

Just before serving, spoon sherbet into a large
punch bowl by heaping tablespoons. Slowly, pour
chilled ginger ale or Sprite over sherbet, stirring
gently. Serve immediately. Makes 1 1/2 quarts.

Mary Johnson

PEANUT BUTTER LOG CANDY

Boil one small potato with jacket on. Mash
potato. Add 1 lb. powdered sugar and mix.
Roll out on wax paper and spread peanut butter
on. Then roll into peanut butter log and
slice in small pieces.

PEANUT BUTTER FUDGE

Mary Johnson

2 cups sugar
1 small can evaporated milk
2 squares chocolate or 4 Tbsp. cocoa
1 tsp. vanilla
1 cup peanut butter
small lump of butter

Boil sugar, milk, chocolate and butter to soft
ball stage. Remove from heat; add vanilla and
peanut butter. Beat until thickens slightly.
Pour on buttered pan. Cut when cool.

HOT POTATO SALAD
Jane Johnson

Ingredients:
6-8 red potatoes (boiled with peeling on)
6 hard boiled eggs
1 lb. bacon (crisp & crumbled)
1 medium onion
Sauce: 2 cups mayonnaise
       6 Tbs. prepared mustard
       1/2 cup sugar
Layer all ingredients.
Then, pour sauce over top.
Cook at 350 until bubbly.

Tropical Hawaiian Wedding Cake
by Geraldine McGowan

1 yellow cake mix cooked in
oblong pan according to
directions
1 large can crushed pineapple,
with juice and 1 c. sugar.
Boil 5 minutes.

When cake comes out of oven
punch holes in it and pour
pineapple mixture over it.

1 large package instant
vanilla pudding mixed
according to package
directions. Pour over
pineapple mixture on cake.
Sprinkle one cup of coconut
over pudding. Cover with
plastic wrap. Refrigerate
over night. Cover with cool
whip and serve.

Cream Puff Cake
By Avalene Dockery

Crust:
1 c. water
1 stick margarine
1/4 t. salt
1 c. plain flour
4 eggs

Boil water and margarine, turn
down to low and add flour and
salt to mixture. Let cool 5
minutes, add eggs (one at a
time) mix until smooth after
each is added. Spread into 9
x 13 pan spreading 1/2 " to
3/4 " up sides of pan. Bake
at 400 degrees for 25 minutes.

Filling:
2 large (5 1/4 oz) pkg.
instant vanilla pudding
3 1/2 c. milk
1 8 oz. cream cheese
1 8 oz. cool whip

Beat cream cheese in a small
bowl, in another bowl beat
pudding with milk then add
cream cheese. Spread on crust
top with cool whip. Drizzle
chocolate syrup over all make
day before serving.

Blueberries in the Snow
Geraldine McGowan

1 large angel food cake
1 c prepared blueberry pie
filling
1 box whipped topping (2
envelopes Dream Whip)
1 c. sugar
1 8 oz. pkg. cream cheese

Soften cream cheese. Mix with
sugar. Mix whipped topping as
directed on package. Add to
mix and mix well. Pour 1/2 of
mixture into oblong pan to
cover bottom. Slice cake in
1/2 inch slices, place cake in
pan. Pour rest of mixture
over cake. Top with pie
filling. Chill 4 hours or
over night.

Broccoli Casserole
Geraldine McGowan

1 small box chopped broccoli
1 can cream of mushroom soup
and 1/2 can water
1 small jar cheese whiz
(melted)
1 1/2 c. minute rice uncooked
1/2 c. onion
1/2 c celery

Pour into a greased or
buttered dish, cut better on
top.
Bake at 350 degrees for 30
minutes.

Oven Stew
Michelle Kerr

1 1/2 lbs. beef, cubed
2 cans Golden Mushroom Soup
1 Tablespoons water
salt and pepper

Place raw beef in 2 quart
casserole dish. Add salt and
pepper to taste. Add soup and
water. Stir together. Bake
at 325 degrees for 2 to 2 1/2
hrs. or until done.

FLUFFY PEANUT BUTTER PIE
Aldine Dockery

8 oz. Cream Cheese
1 cup powdered sugar
1/2 cup peanut butter
1/2 teaspoon vanilla
1 small container Cool Whip
Chopped pecans or peanuts
1 9" Graham Cracker Pie Crust

With a mixer, mix all ingredients except
for Cool Whip, vanilla, and nuts.
Fold in Cool Whip and vanilla.
Pour into crust. Sprinkle with nuts. Chill.

Seven Layer Cookies
By Pearlie McQueary

1/4 lb. butter (1/2 c. or 1
stick)
1 c. graham crackers
1 16 oz. bag butterscotch
chips
1 16 oz. bag chocolate chips
1 c. coconut
1 c. chopped pecans
1 14 oz. can eagle brand milk

Melt butter mix with cracker
crumbs, line 9 x 13 " pan.
Add coconut, butterscotch
chips, chocolate chips and
nuts. Spread eagle brand milk
on top. Bake 25-30 minutes at
360 degrees.

HOT SPAM SALAD
Rita Gosser

Ingredients:

One large can of Spam (grated)
6 oz. grated "Hot" Cheese
One small - medium onion (chopped)
1 heaping Tbs. Pickle relish
3 heaping Tbs. Mayonnaise.

Stir all ingredients together.
Serve on crackers.

Country Chicken Casserole
By Barbara Wilson

5 oz. spaghetti
1/2 box frozen mixed
vegetables. or 1 small can
peas & carrots
8 oz. velveeta cheese
1/8 c. mayonnaise
1/2 c. milk
1 can chicken or turkey

Cook spaghetti and mixed
vegetables separately.
Combine cheese and milk. Cook
until melted . Add mayo and
meat, stir. Drain spaghetti
and vegetables. Put into
casserole dish. Pour cheese
mixture over this. Mix.
Bake in oven or microwave
until hot.

Pistachio Cake
JoAnn Conner

1 box white cake mix
3/4 cup vegetable oil
3/4 cup water
4 eggs
1 3 oz Pistachio Instant
pudding
1/2 c. chopped nuts

Glaze:
1/2 cup hot water
1 lbs. butter, melted
2 cups powdered sugar
1/2 tsp. vanilla

Cake: Combine cake mix, oil,
water, eggs, and pudding mix.
Beat about 4 minutes at medium
speed. Pour into greased and
floured 13 x 9 pan. Sprinkle
top with nuts. Bake at 350
degrees for 35 to 40 minutes.

Glaze:
Place water, butter, powdered
sugar and vanilla in small
bowl and beat with a fork.
While cake is still hot punch
holes with a fork over entire
top. Spoon icing over cake
allowing it to run down into
holes. Pry holes open if
necessary to insure that the
icing runs into cake. Stays
moist.

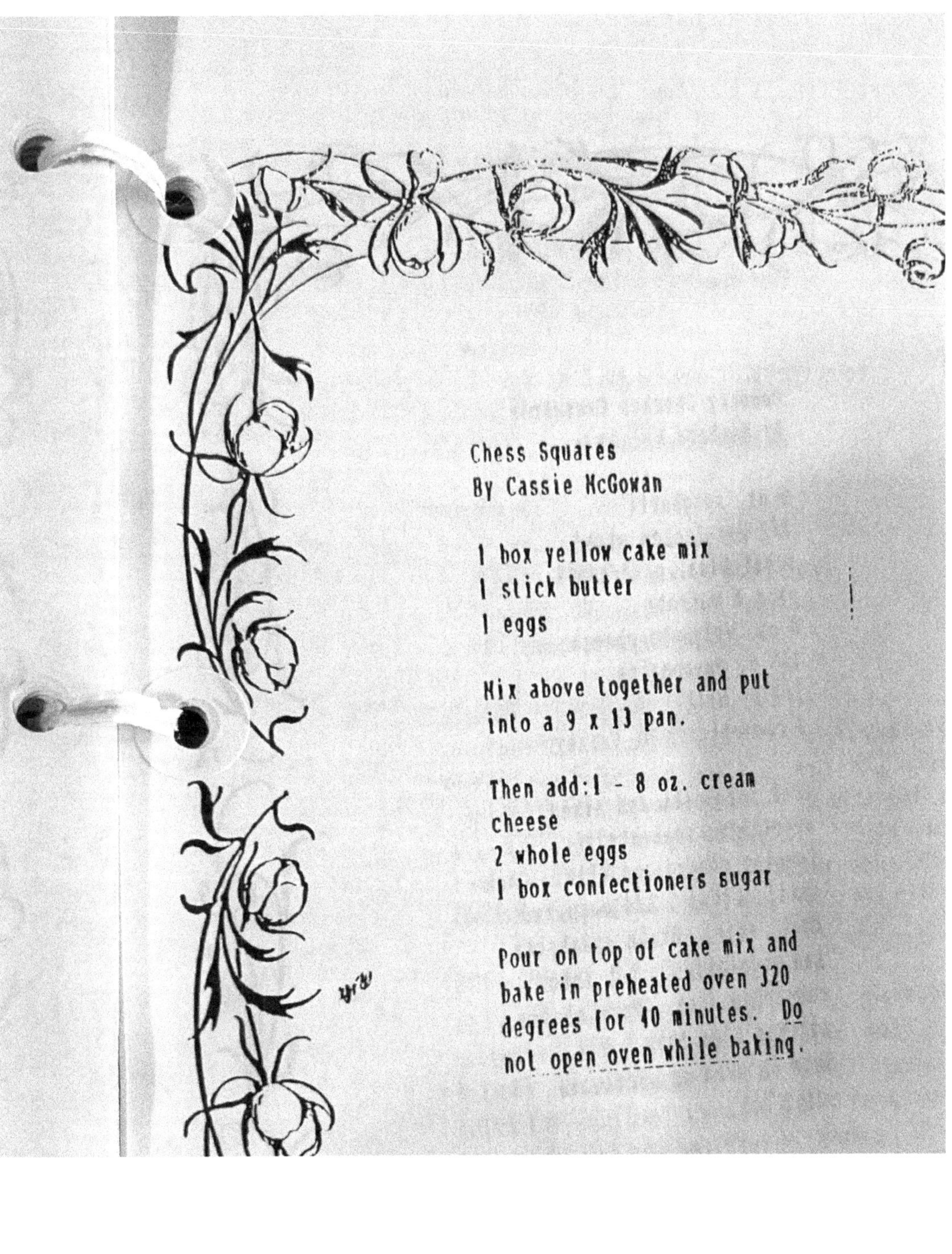

Chess Squares
By Cassie McGowan

1 box yellow cake mix
1 stick butter
1 eggs

Mix above together and put
into a 9 x 13 pan.

Then add:1 - 8 oz. cream
cheese
2 whole eggs
1 box confectioners sugar

Pour on top of cake mix and
bake in preheated oven 320
degrees for 40 minutes. Do
not open oven while baking.

Baked Spaghetti
Jo Ann Conner

1 cup chopped onion
1 cup chopped green pepper
1 Tbs. butter or margarine
1 can (28 oz) tomatoes, with
liquid, cut up
8 oz tomato sauce
1 can (4 oz) mushroom stems
and pieces drained
1 can (2 1/4 oz) sliced rip
olives, drained, optional
2 tsp. dried oregano
1 lb. ground beef, browned and
drained,
12 oz. spaghetti, cooked and
drained
2 cups (8 oz) shredded cheddar
cheese
1 can (10 3/4 oz) condensed
cream of mushroom soup
undiluted
1/4 cup water
1/4 cup grated Parmesan cheese

In a large skillet, saute
onion and green pepper in
butter until tender, all
tomatoes, sauce, mushrooms,
olives and oregano. Add
ground beef if desired.
Simmer, uncovered for 10
minutes. Place half of the
spaghetti in a greased 13 x 9
baking dish. Top with half of
the vegetable mixture.
Sprinkle with 1 cup of cheddar
cheese, repeat layers, mix the
soup and water until smooth;
pour over casserole. Sprinkle
with Parmesan cheese. Bake
uncovered at 350 degrees for
30-35 minutes or until heated
through. Yield-12 servings.
Leftovers freeze well for a
quick meal later in week.

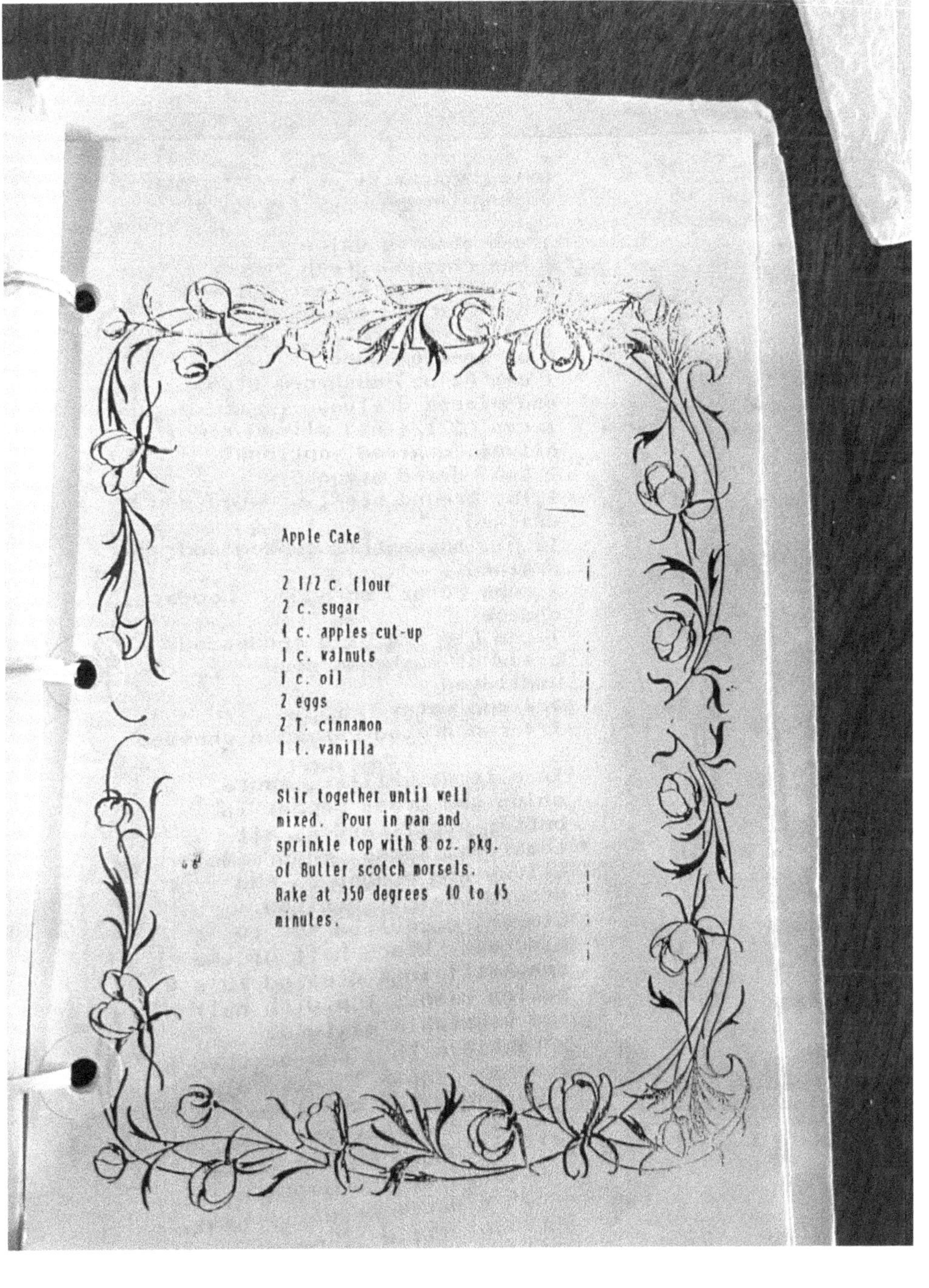

Apple Cake

2 1/2 c. flour
2 c. sugar
4 c. apples cut-up
1 c. walnuts
1 c. oil
2 eggs
2 T. cinnamon
1 t. vanilla

Stir together until well
mixed. Pour in pan and
sprinkle top with 8 oz. pkg.
of Butter scotch morsels.
Bake at 350 degrees 40 to 45
minutes.

Honey Bun Cake
      Pearl Roy

1 Box yellow cake mix (Duncan
Hines)
4 eggs
8 oz. sour cream
3/4 cup of vegetable oil

      Pour half in greased pan
then sprinkle mixture of
  2 cups of brown sugar
  2 T. cinnamon (more if
needed)
Pour remaining cake mix & take
fingers to spread.
  Bake at 350 degrees for 25-30
minutes.
While cake is baking mix
frosting.
3 cups of powdered sugar
2 t. vanilla
1 cup of milk
Pour over cake while hot.
Punch holes incake so frosting
will go into cake.

Oatmeal Pie
By Maxine Hadley

2 beaten eggs
3/4 c. sugar
1/2 c. flaked coconut
3/4 c. oatmeal
1/2 c. melted butter
3/4 dark syrup
pinch of salt

Mix well pour into unbaked
shell and bake in 350 degrees
oven about 30 to 40 minutes or
until custard begins to set.

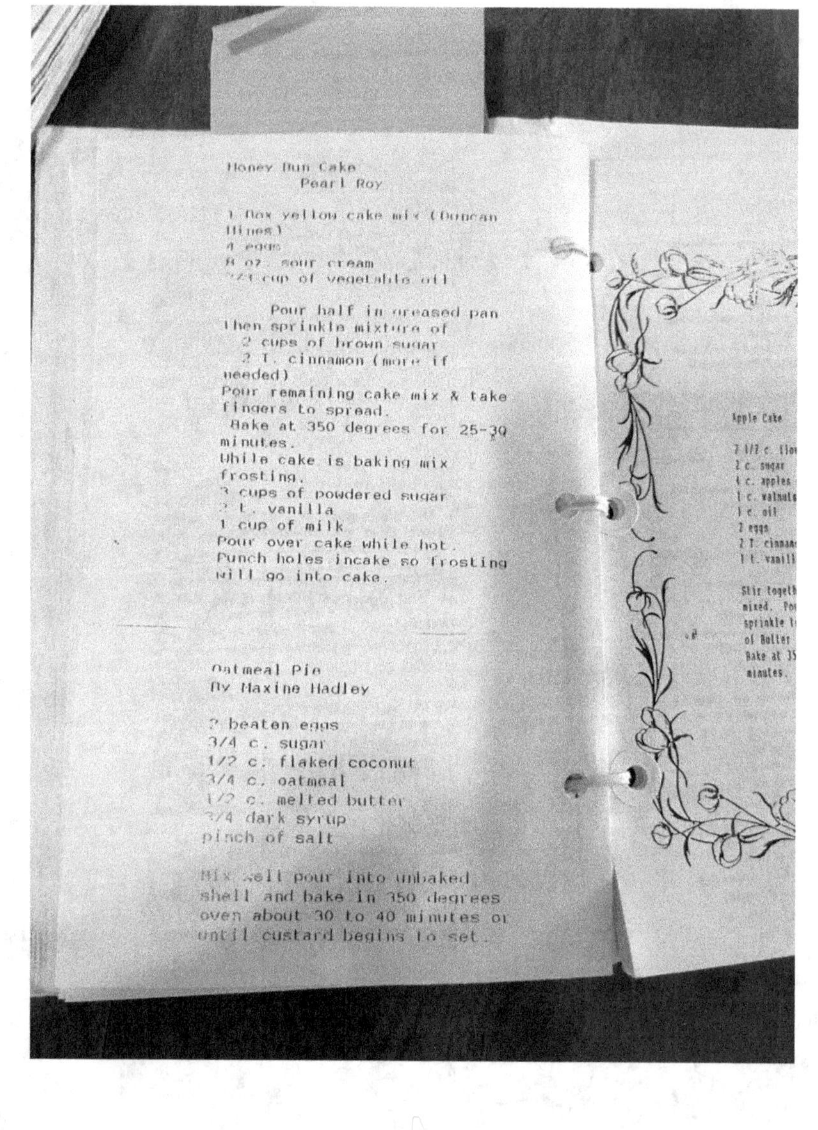

Apple Cake

2 1/2 c. flour
2 c. sugar
4 c. apples
1 c. walnuts
1 c. oil
2 eggs
2 T. cinnamon
1 t. vanilla

Stir togeth
mixed. Po
sprinkle t
of Butter
Bake at 35
minutes.

Lola's Never Fail Pie Crust
By Sallie C. Dunbar

1 c. lard
1/2 c. of boiling water
1/4 t. baking powder
pinch of salt 2 1/2 c. of all
purpose flour

Pour boiling water over lard
and stir until dissolved, add
remaining ingredients. Chill
thoroughly. Keeps in covered
dish in refrigerator for
weeks. Home rendered lard is
ideal

Sausage Balls
By Doris Dick

1 lb. sausage
1-8oz. jar of cheez whiz
2 cups Bisquick

Mix at room temperature. Bake
at 350 degrees until done.

Strawberry Pie
By Doris Dick

1 small box strawberry jello
1 small can crushed pineapple
1 cup white sugar
Mix together and cook until it
gets thick (stir often) let
cool

Have 1 large can carnation
cream chilled. Beat it with
electric mixer until it gets
thick, add 1 cup of pecans and
the above mixture put into
graham cracker crust. Makes 2
pies.

Lola's Never Fail Pie Crust
By Sallie C. Dunbar

1 c. lard
1/2 c. of boiling water
1/2 t. baking powder
pinch of salt 2 1/2 c. of all
purpose flour

Pour boiling water over lard
and stir until dissolved, add
remaining ingredients. Chill
thoroughly. Keeps in covered
dish in refrigerator for
weeks. Home rendered lard is
ideal.

Sausage Balls
By Doris Dick

1 lb. sausage
1-8oz. jar of cheez whiz
2 cups Bisquick

Mix at room temperature. Bake
at 350 degrees until done.

Strawberry Pie
By Doris Dick

1 small box strawberry Jello
1 small can crushed pineapple
1 cup white sugar
Mix together and cook until it
gets thick (stir often) let
cool.

Have 1 large can carnation
cream chilled. Beat it with
electric mixer until it gets
thick, add 1 cup of pecans and
the above mixture put into
graham cracker crust. Makes 2
pies.

Sloppy Joe Casserole
Tracy Popplewell

1 lb. ground beef (browned)
1 pkg. sloppy joe seasoning
15 oz. can tomato sauce
2 cans cresent rolls
1 pkg. mozzarella cheese
slices or 1 1/2 c. shredded

Mix together browned ground
beef, sloppy joe seasoning and
tomato sauce in skillet. In
greased 9 x 13 casserole dish,
lay out one can of the rolls
on bottom of dish. Add beef
mixture, then cheese. top with
second can of rolls. Cover
with foil to bake.
     Bake at 350 degrees for
30 minutes, remove foil, bake
for 10-15 minutes until golden
brown.

Meat Loaf
By Maxine Hadley

1 1/2 lb. ground beef
1 medium onion, chopped
1/4 t. pepper
3/4 c. oats
2 t. salt
2 eggs
1 c. tomato juice

Mix all ingredients. Shape
into loaf. Bake at 350
degrees for one hour.

Sugar Less Fruit Salad
By Avalene Dockery

2 cans lite fruit cocktail
1 can unsweetened crushed
pineapple
1 large orange peeled & diced
1 large apple peeled & diced
1 pkg. sugar free instant
vanilla pudding mix
1 pkg. sugar free strawberry
gelatin

Mix together first four
ingredients. Sprinkle pudding
and gelatin over mixture. Mix
well and cover. Refrigerate
over night before serving.

Texas Sheet Cake
By Marie Popplewell

2 c. sugar
2 c. self-rising flour
2 sticks margarine
1 c. water
4 T. cocoa
1/2 c. buttermilk
2 eggs
1 t. soda

Place flour and sugar in
mixing bowl. In heavy pan,
place butter, water, and
cocoa, bring to a boil or
until butter melts. Pour into
dry ingredients, mix and then
add buttermilk, eggs, and
soda, blend well. Mixture
will be thin. Bake in sheet
type pan at 375 degrees F.
about 17 to 20 minutes. This
is slightly underdone. Remove
from oven and frost
immediately with

Butter Nut Frosting
1 c. Sugar
1 stick Butter
1 T. Cocoa
3 T. Karo Syrup
1/3 c. evaporated milk
2 c. powdered sugar
2 T. Crisco
1 c. chopped nuts

Place in sauce pan, sugar,
butter, cocoa, syrup, and
milk, boil about 5 min. until
sugar is dissolved pour into
bowl and mix well with the
powdered sugar, crisco and
nuts. Pour over hot cake.

Bread Pudding
By Darlene Vaught

3 c. bread cubes (about 3-4
slices)
3 eggs
1/2 c. sugar
1 3/4 c. milk
1 c. boiling water
1/2 t. vanilla

Place bread in a buttered
baking dish. Beat eggs. Add
sugar, and milk. Stir in
vanilla. Pour over bread.
Bake 45 min. to 1 hr. on 350.

Tangy Butter Sauce

1/2 c. butter creamed
1 c. powdered sugar-sifted
Mix until fluffy-set aside
Boil until thick and clear: 1
T. cornstarch
1 c. water
Add above mixture then add 1
T. lemon juice
1 1/2 t. vanilla
Serve warm over pudding or
rice. You may add cinnamon
and raisins if you like.

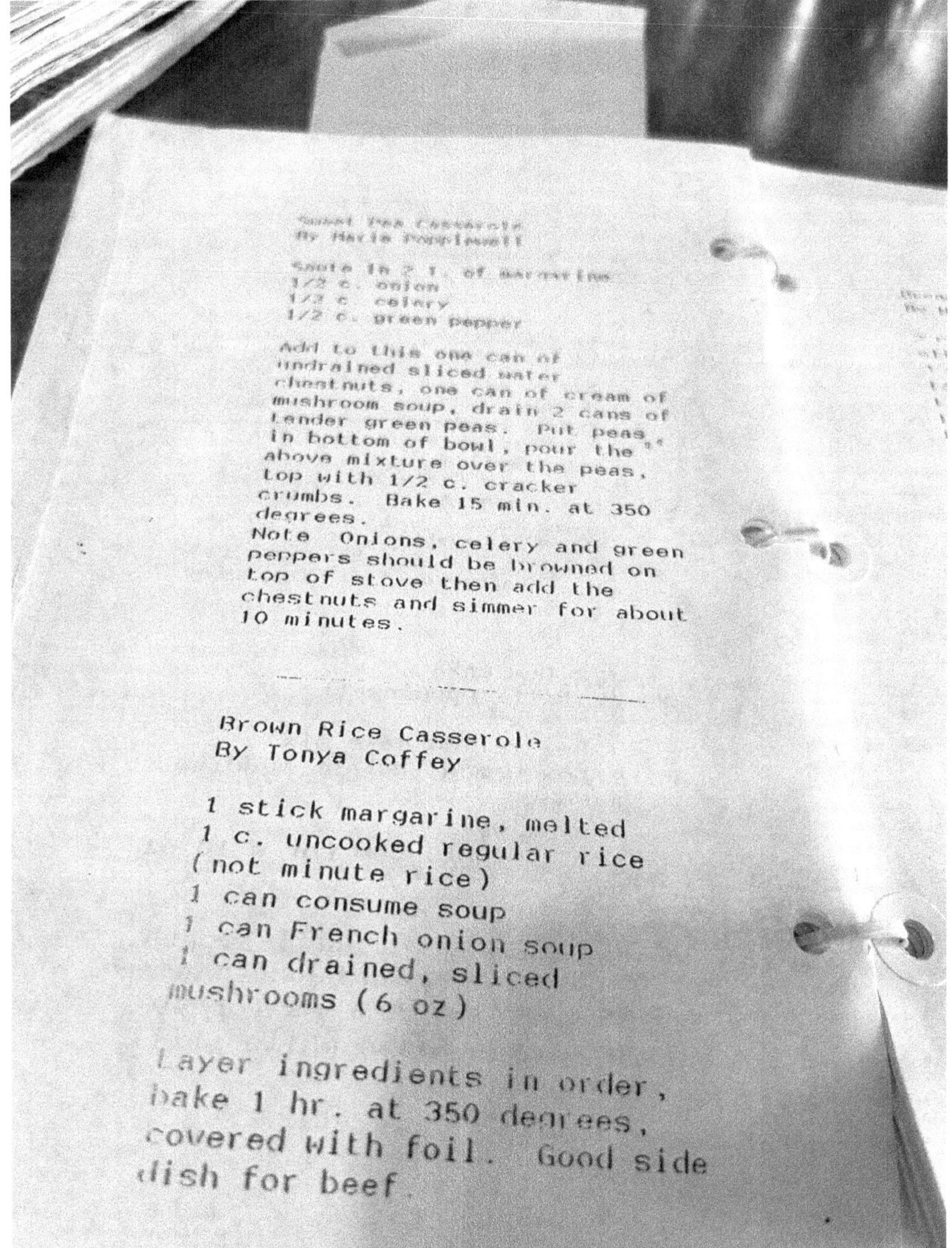

Sweet Pea Casserole
By Maria Popplewell

Saute in 2 T. of margarine
1/2 c. onion
1/2 c. celery
1/2 c. green pepper

Add to this one can of
undrained sliced water
chestnuts, one can of cream of
mushroom soup, drain 2 cans of
tender green peas. Put peas
in bottom of bowl, pour the
above mixture over the peas,
top with 1/2 c. cracker
crumbs. Bake 15 min. at 350
degrees.
Note Onions, celery and green
peppers should be browned on
top of stove then add the
chestnuts and simmer for about
10 minutes.

Brown Rice Casserole
By Tonya Coffey

1 stick margarine, melted
1 c. uncooked regular rice
(not minute rice)
1 can consume soup
1 can French onion soup
1 can drained, sliced
mushrooms (6 oz)

Layer ingredients in order,
bake 1 hr. at 350 degrees,
covered with foil. Good side
dish for beef.

Coconut Pecan Bars
By Betty Popplewell

3/4 c. oil
2 eggs
3/4 c. powdered sugar
1 1/2 c. self rising flour
1 t. vanilla
1 c. nuts (Pecans)
1 c. coconut

Mix all together. pour in
greased 13 x 9 cake pan. Bake
at 350 degrees for 15 minutes.

Mt. Dew Cake
By Betty Popplewell

1 box yellow cake mix
1 box Lemon Instant pudding
4 eggs
3/4 c. oil
1 1/4 c. Mt. Dew (or a 10 oz
can)

Mix with mixer until smooth,
pour in greased bundt pan and
bake at 350 degrees for 40
minutes. Glaze while still
warm.

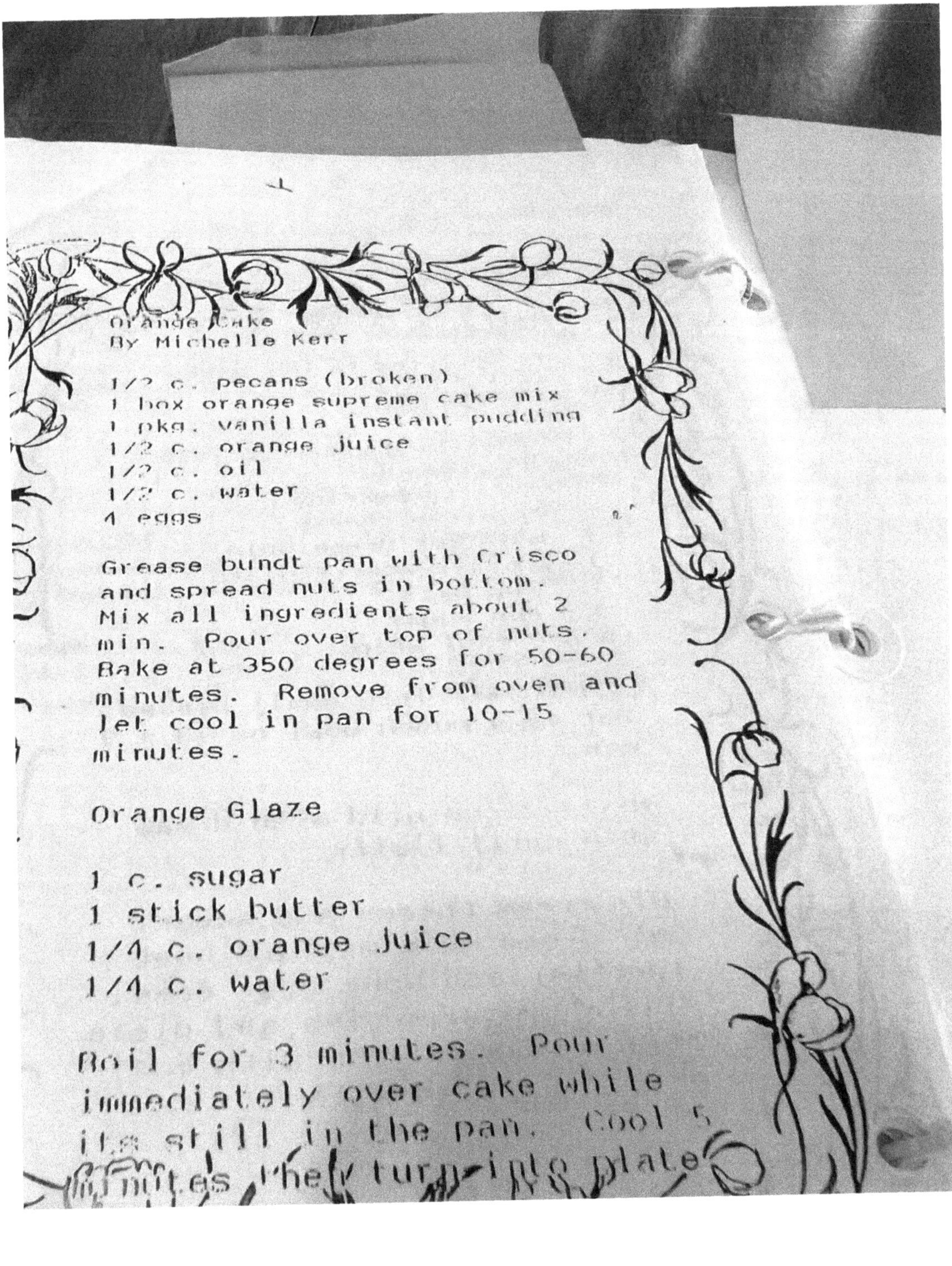

Orange Cake
By Michelle Kerr

1/2 c. pecans (broken)
1 box orange supreme cake mix
1 pkg. vanilla instant pudding
1/2 c. orange juice
1/2 c. oil
1/2 c. water
4 eggs

Grease bundt pan with Crisco
and spread nuts in bottom.
Mix all ingredients about 2
min. Pour over top of nuts.
Bake at 350 degrees for 50-60
minutes. Remove from oven and
let cool in pan for 10-15
minutes.

Orange Glaze

1 c. sugar
1 stick butter
1/4 c. orange juice
1/4 c. water

Boil for 3 minutes. Pour
immediately over cake while
its still in the pan. Cool 5
minutes then turn into plate

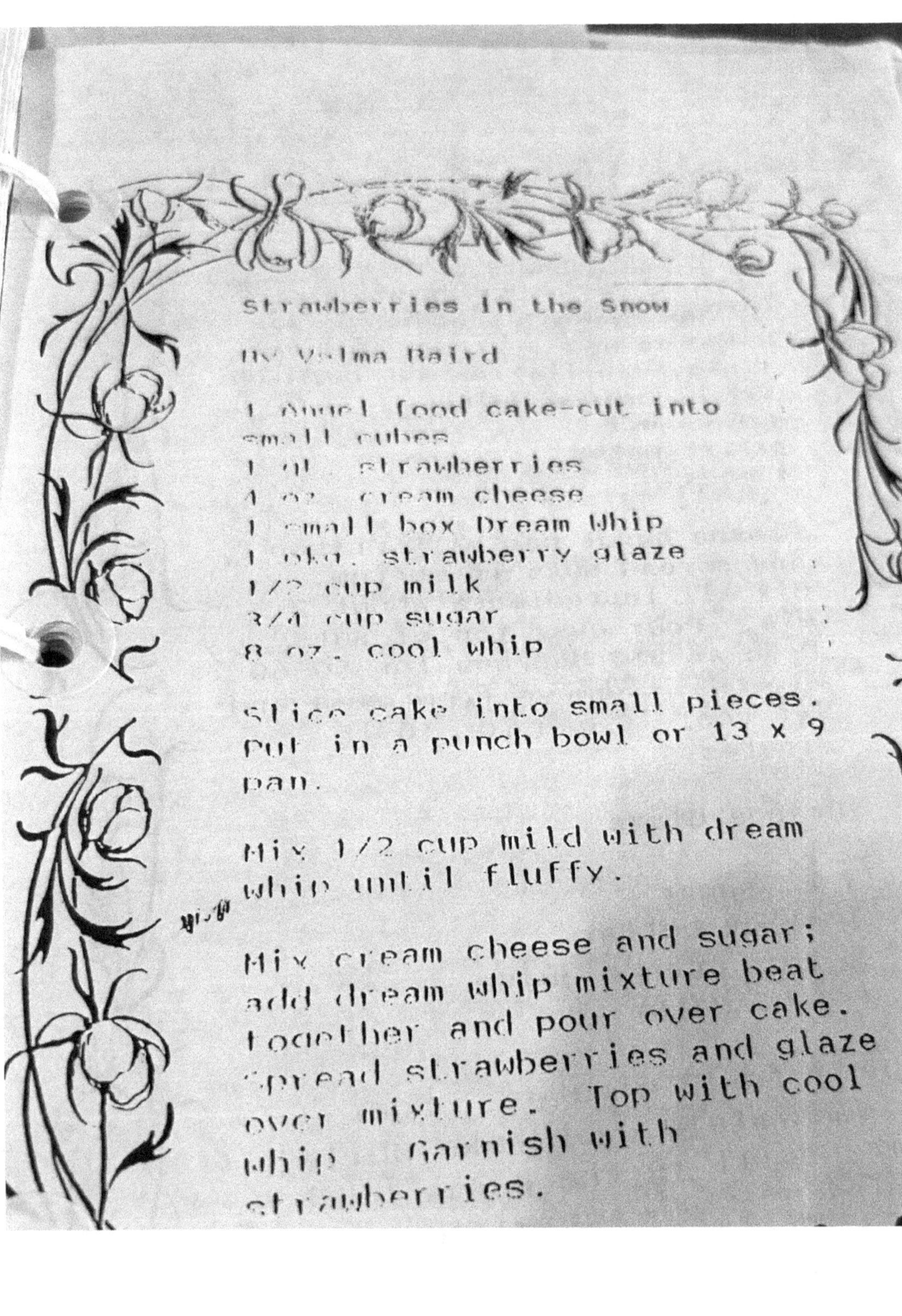

Strawberries In the Snow

By Velma Baird

1 Angel food cake-cut into
small cubes
1 qt. strawberries
1 oz. cream cheese
1 small box Dream Whip
1 pkg. strawberry glaze
1/2 cup milk
3/4 cup sugar
8 oz. cool whip

Slice cake into small pieces.
Put in a punch bowl or 13 x 9
pan.

Mix 1/2 cup mild with dream
whip until fluffy.

Mix cream cheese and sugar;
add dream whip mixture beat
together and pour over cake.
Spread strawberries and glaze
over mixture. Top with cool
whip. Garnish with
strawberries.

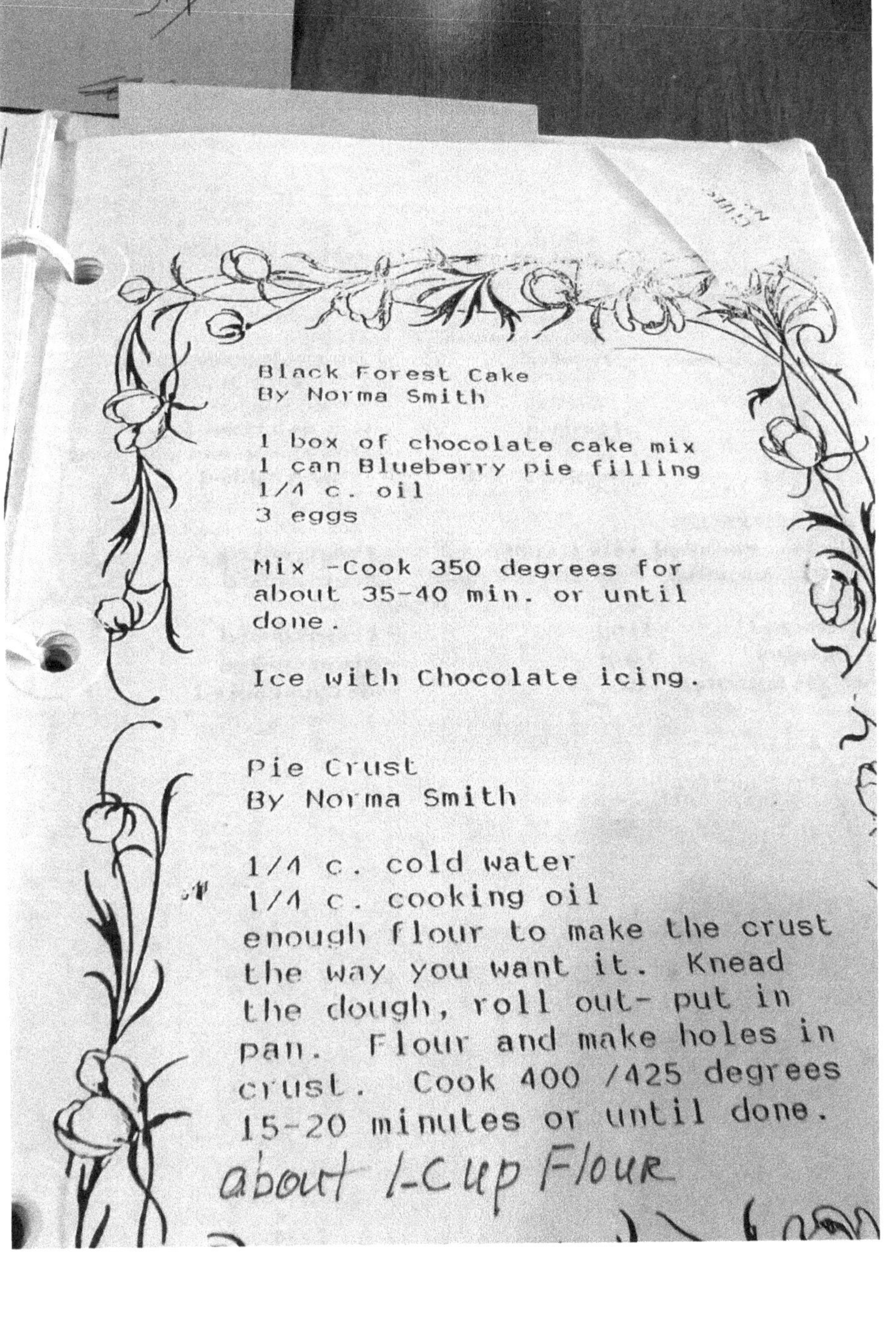

Black Forest Cake
By Norma Smith

1 box of chocolate cake mix
1 can Blueberry pie filling
1/4 c. oil
3 eggs

Mix -Cook 350 degrees for about 35-40 min. or until done.

Ice with Chocolate icing.

Pie Crust
By Norma Smith

1/4 c. cold water
1/4 c. cooking oil
enough flour to make the crust the way you want it. Knead the dough, roll out- put in pan. Flour and make holes in crust. Cook 400 /425 degrees 15-20 minutes or until done.

about 1-Cup Flour

OZARK PUDDING

8 Tbs. flour

1 1/2 C. sugar (1 C. white, 1/2 C.
brown)

1 C. nuts

1 Tsp. salt

1 Tsp. vanilla

1 Tsp. baking powder

1 C. apples (chopped)

Mix up and bake until brown,

about 25 or 30 min.

Modine Vaught

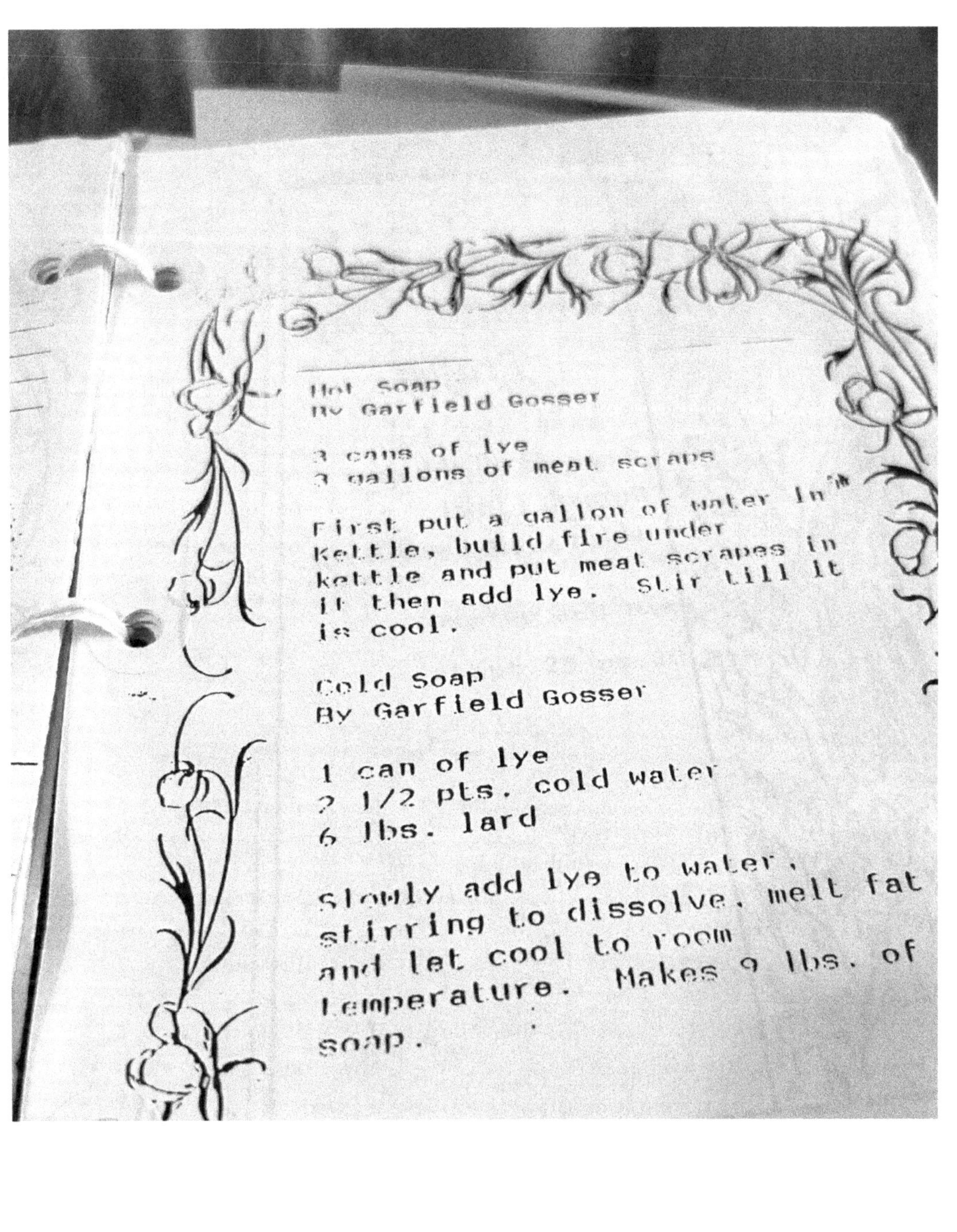

Hot Soap
By Garfield Gosser

3 cans of lye
3 gallons of meat scraps

First put a gallon of water in
kettle, build fire under
kettle and put meat scrapes in
it then add lye. Stir till it
is cool.

Cold Soap
By Garfield Gosser

1 can of lye
2 1/2 pts. cold water
6 lbs. lard

Slowly add lye to water,
stirring to dissolve. Melt fat
and let cool to room
temperature. Makes 9 lbs. of
soap.

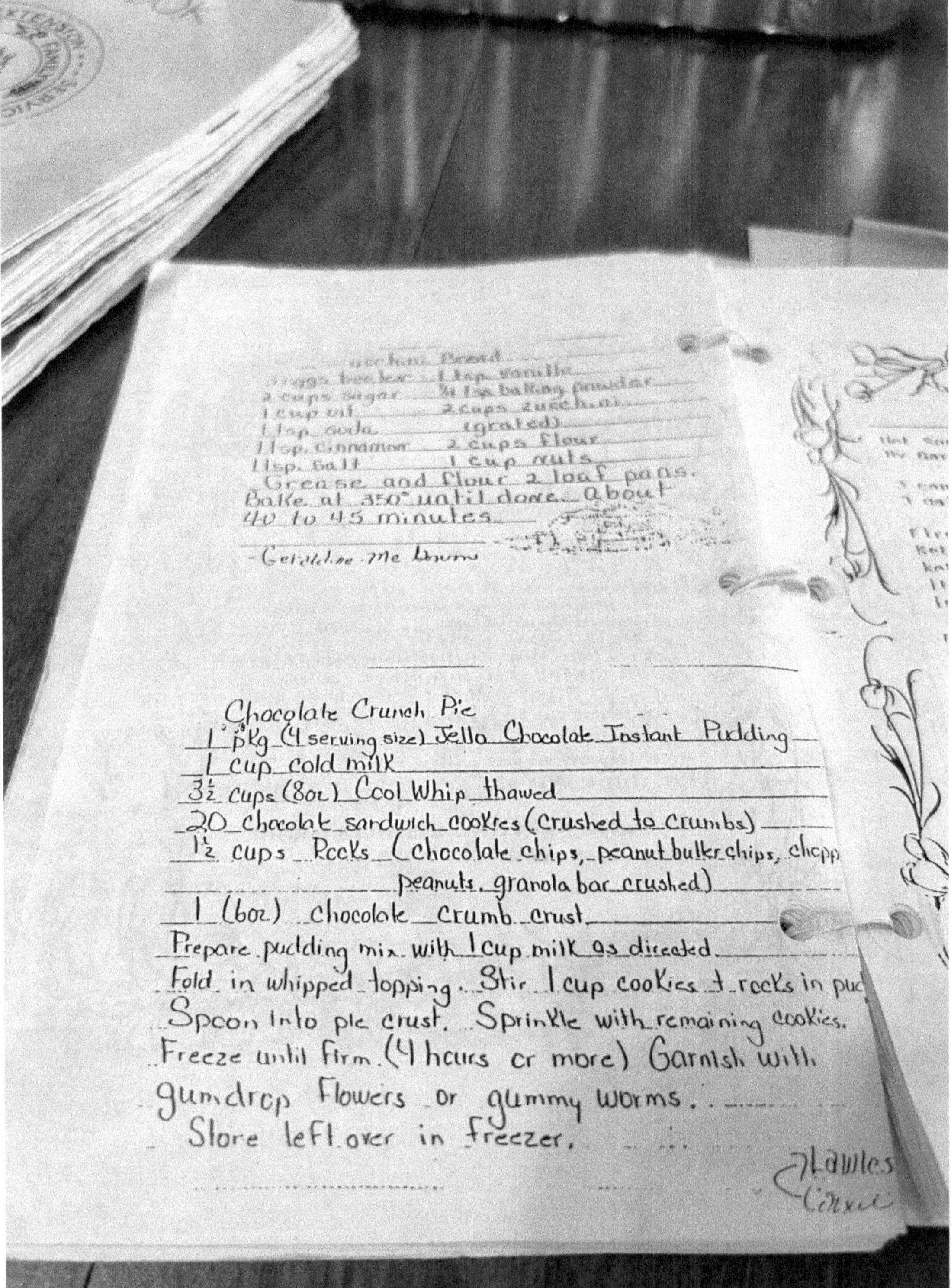

...cchini Bread

3 eggs beaten	1 tsp. vanilla
2 cups sugar	¼ tsp. baking powder
1 cup oil	2 cups zucchini
1 tsp. soda	(grated)
1 tsp. cinnamon	2 cups flour
1 tsp. salt	1 cup nuts

Grease and flour 2 loaf pans.
Bake at 350° until done. About
40 to 45 minutes

— Geraldine McBroom

Chocolate Crunch Pie
1 pkg (4 serving size) Jello Chocolate Instant Pudding
1 cup cold milk
3½ cups (8oz) Cool Whip thawed
20 chocolate sandwich cookies (crushed to crumbs)
1½ cups Rocks (chocolate chips, peanut butter chips, chopp
                    peanuts, granola bar crushed)
1 (6oz) chocolate crumb crust
Prepare pudding mix with 1 cup milk as directed
Fold in whipped topping. Stir 1 cup cookies + rocks in pud
Spoon into pie crust. Sprinkle with remaining cookies.
Freeze until firm (4 hours or more) Garnish with
gumdrop flowers or gummy worms.
Store leftover in freezer.

Lawles Corner

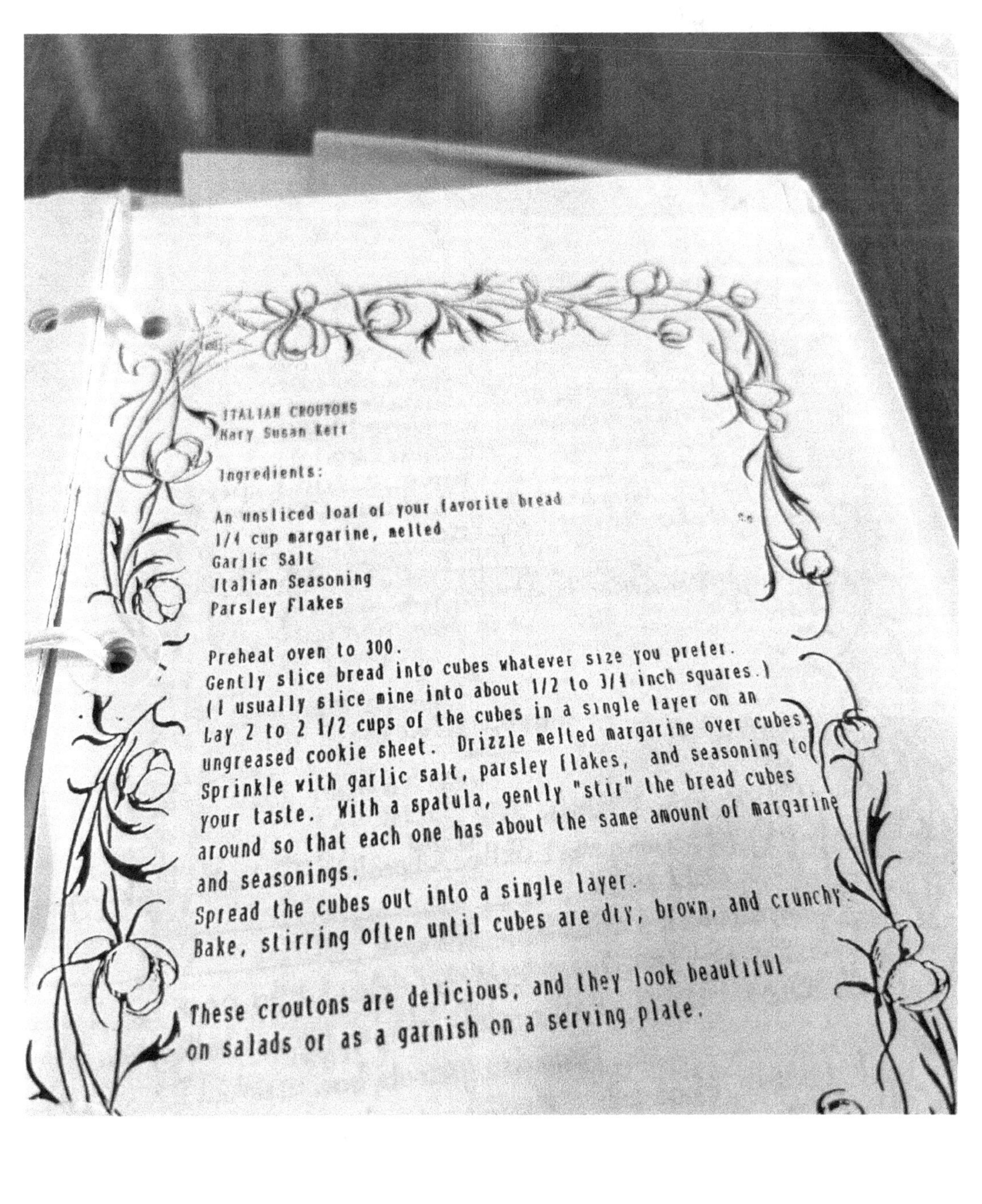

ITALIAN CROUTONS
Mary Susan Kerr

Ingredients:

An unsliced loaf of your favorite bread
1/4 cup margarine, melted
Garlic Salt
Italian Seasoning
Parsley Flakes

Preheat oven to 300.
Gently slice bread into cubes whatever size you prefer.
(I usually slice mine into about 1/2 to 3/4 inch squares.)
Lay 2 to 2 1/2 cups of the cubes in a single layer on an
ungreased cookie sheet. Drizzle melted margarine over cubes.
Sprinkle with garlic salt, parsley flakes, and seasoning to
your taste. With a spatula, gently "stir" the bread cubes
around so that each one has about the same amount of margarine
and seasonings.
Spread the cubes out into a single layer.
Bake, stirring often until cubes are dry, brown, and crunchy.

These croutons are delicious, and they look beautiful
on salads or as a garnish on a serving plate.

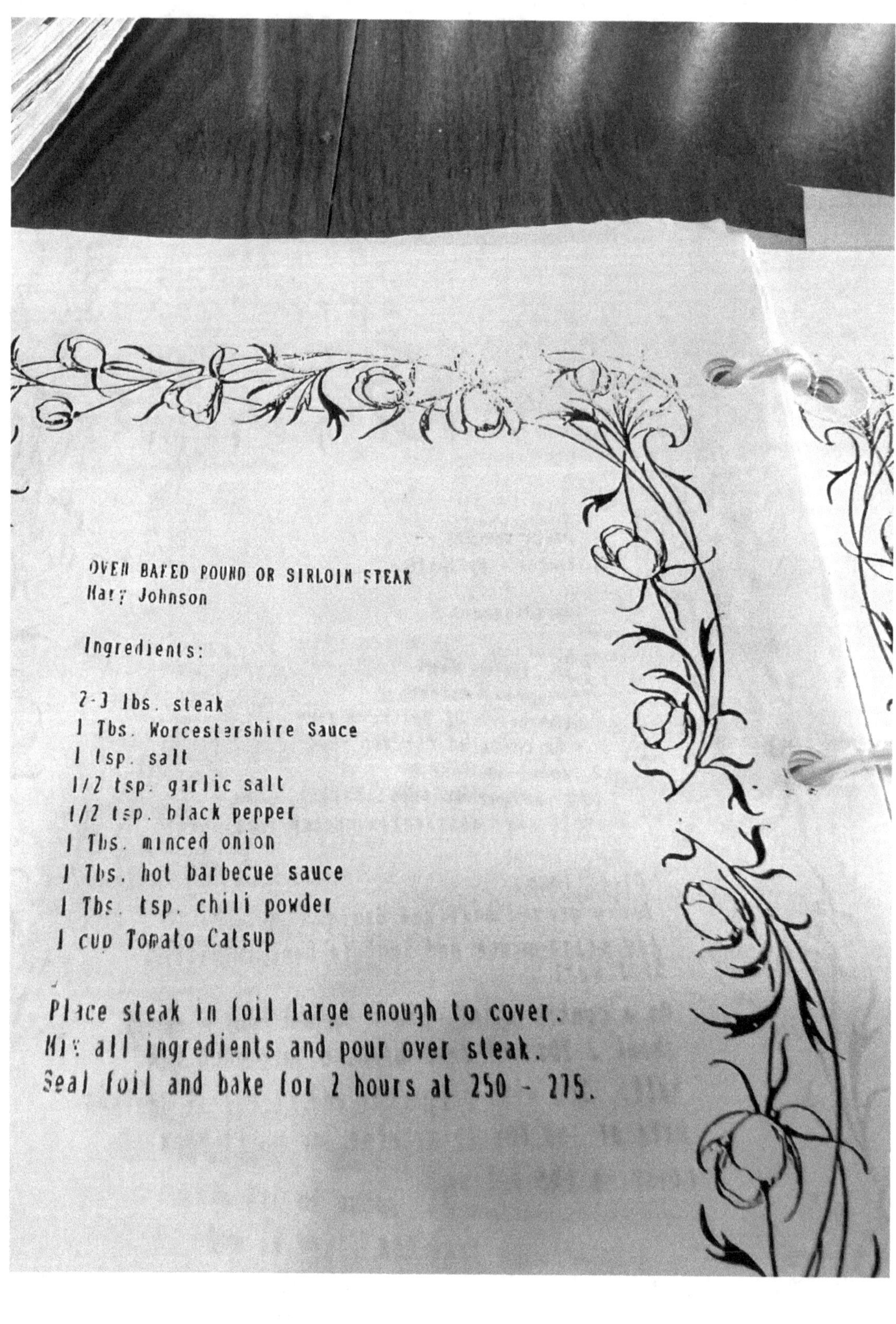

OVEN BAKED ROUND OR SIRLOIN STEAK
Mary Johnson

Ingredients:

2-3 lbs. steak
1 Tbs. Worcestershire Sauce
1 tsp. salt
1/2 tsp. garlic salt
1/2 tsp. black pepper
1 Tbs. minced onion
1 Tbs. hot barbecue sauce
1 Tbs. tsp. chili powder
1 cup Tomato Catsup

Place steak in foil large enough to cover.
Mix all ingredients and pour over steak.
Seal foil and bake for 2 hours at 250 - 275.

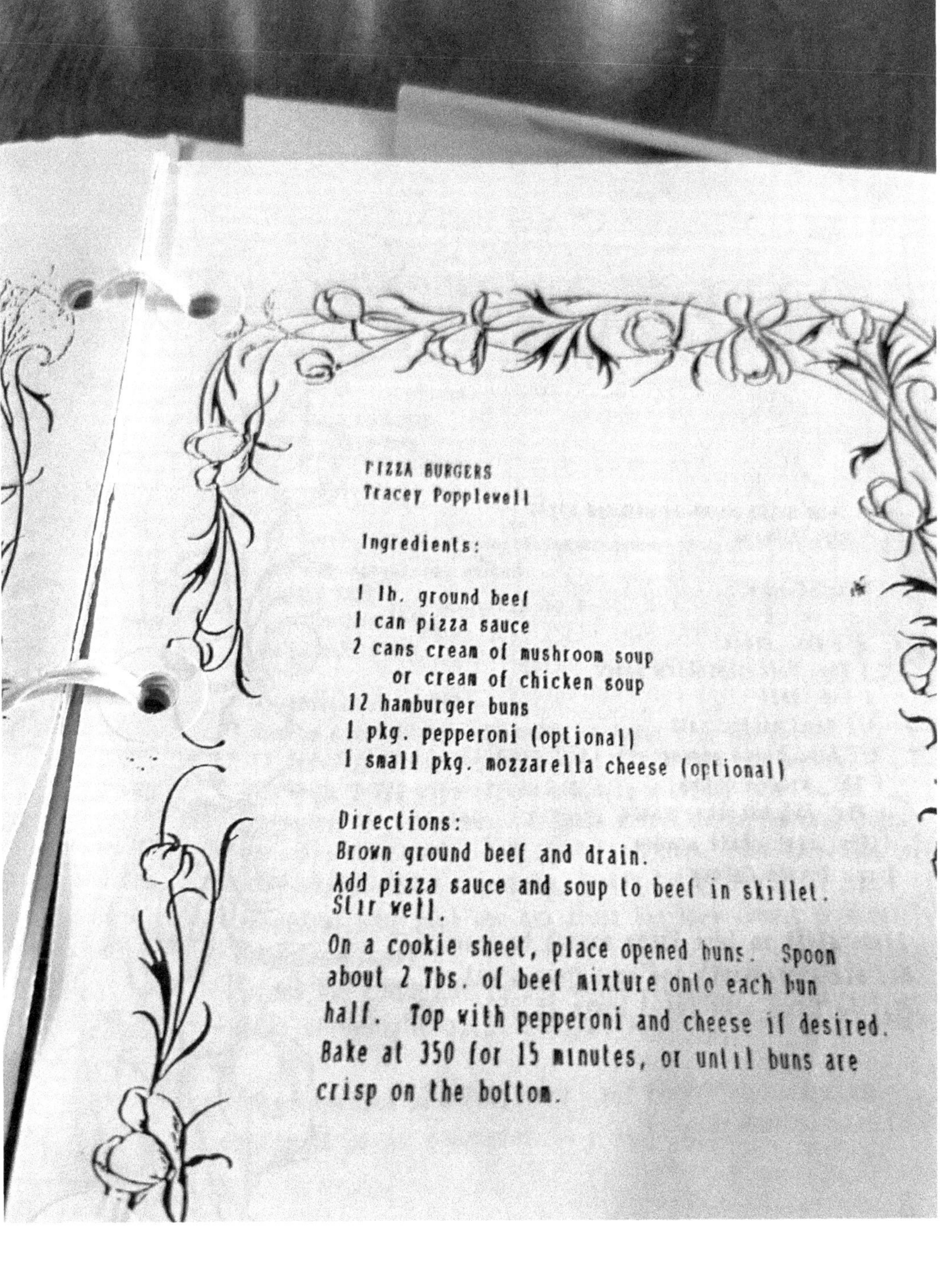

PIZZA BURGERS
Tracey Popplewell

Ingredients:

1 lb. ground beef
1 can pizza sauce
2 cans cream of mushroom soup
    or cream of chicken soup
12 hamburger buns
1 pkg. pepperoni (optional)
1 small pkg. mozzarella cheese (optional)

Directions:
Brown ground beef and drain.
Add pizza sauce and soup to beef in skillet.
Stir well.

On a cookie sheet, place opened buns. Spoon
about 2 Tbs. of beef mixture onto each bun
half. Top with pepperoni and cheese if desired.
Bake at 350 for 15 minutes, or until buns are
crisp on the bottom.

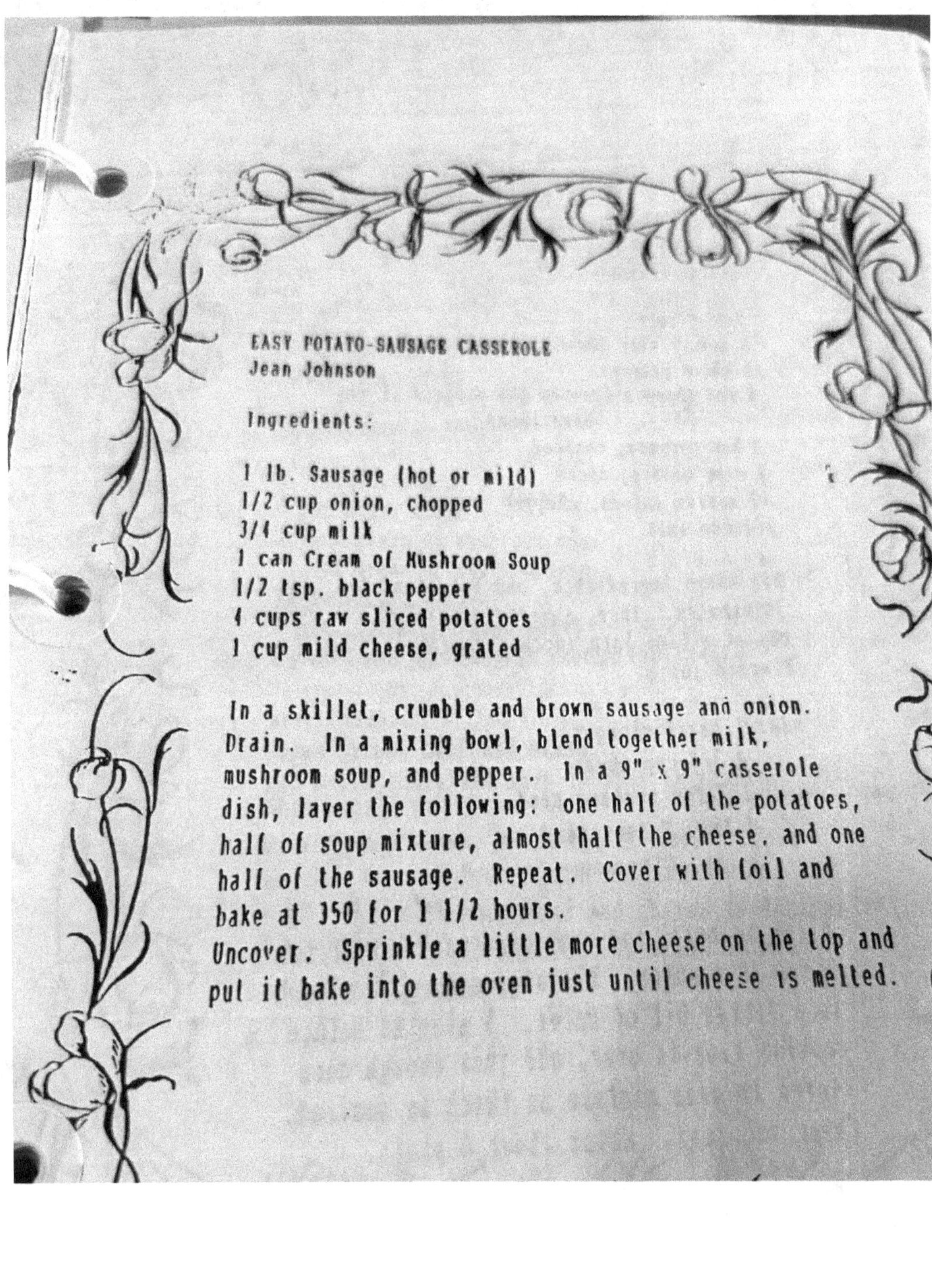

EASY POTATO-SAUSAGE CASSEROLE
Jean Johnson

Ingredients:

1 lb. Sausage (hot or mild)
1/2 cup onion, chopped
3/4 cup milk
1 can Cream of Mushroom Soup
1/2 tsp. black pepper
4 cups raw sliced potatoes
1 cup mild cheese, grated

In a skillet, crumble and brown sausage and onion.
Drain. In a mixing bowl, blend together milk,
mushroom soup, and pepper. In a 9" x 9" casserole
dish, layer the following: one half of the potatoes,
half of soup mixture, almost half the cheese, and one
half of the sausage. Repeat. Cover with foil and
bake at 350 for 1 1/2 hours.
Uncover. Sprinkle a little more cheese on the top and
put it bake into the oven just until cheese is melted.

1 3/4 C. flour   48 Hershey Kisses
1/3 C. brown sugar
1/2 C. butter
1 egg
1 tsp. vanilla
1/2 C. sugar
1/2 C. peanut butter
2 Tbl. milk

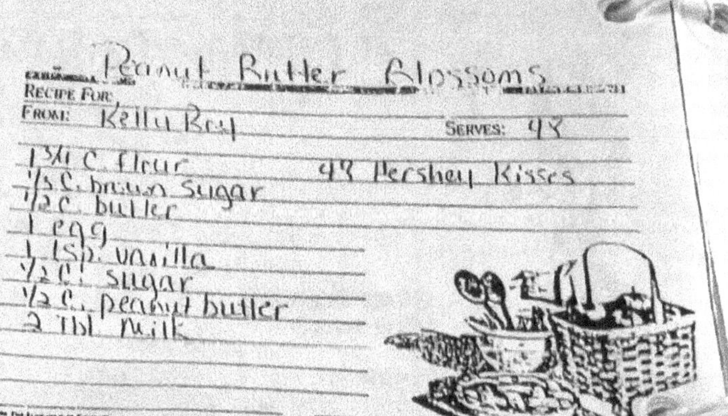

- Combine all ingredients but Hershey Kisses and mix on low with mixer until doughy. Shape into round balls
- (jackball - walnut size) and roll in extra sugar. Place on ungreased cookie sheet and bake at 375° for 10-12 minutes.
- Immediately top with Kisses, press down until cookie cracks around candy. This Kiss will completely melt, but hold its shape. Do not touch it, they will firm back up.

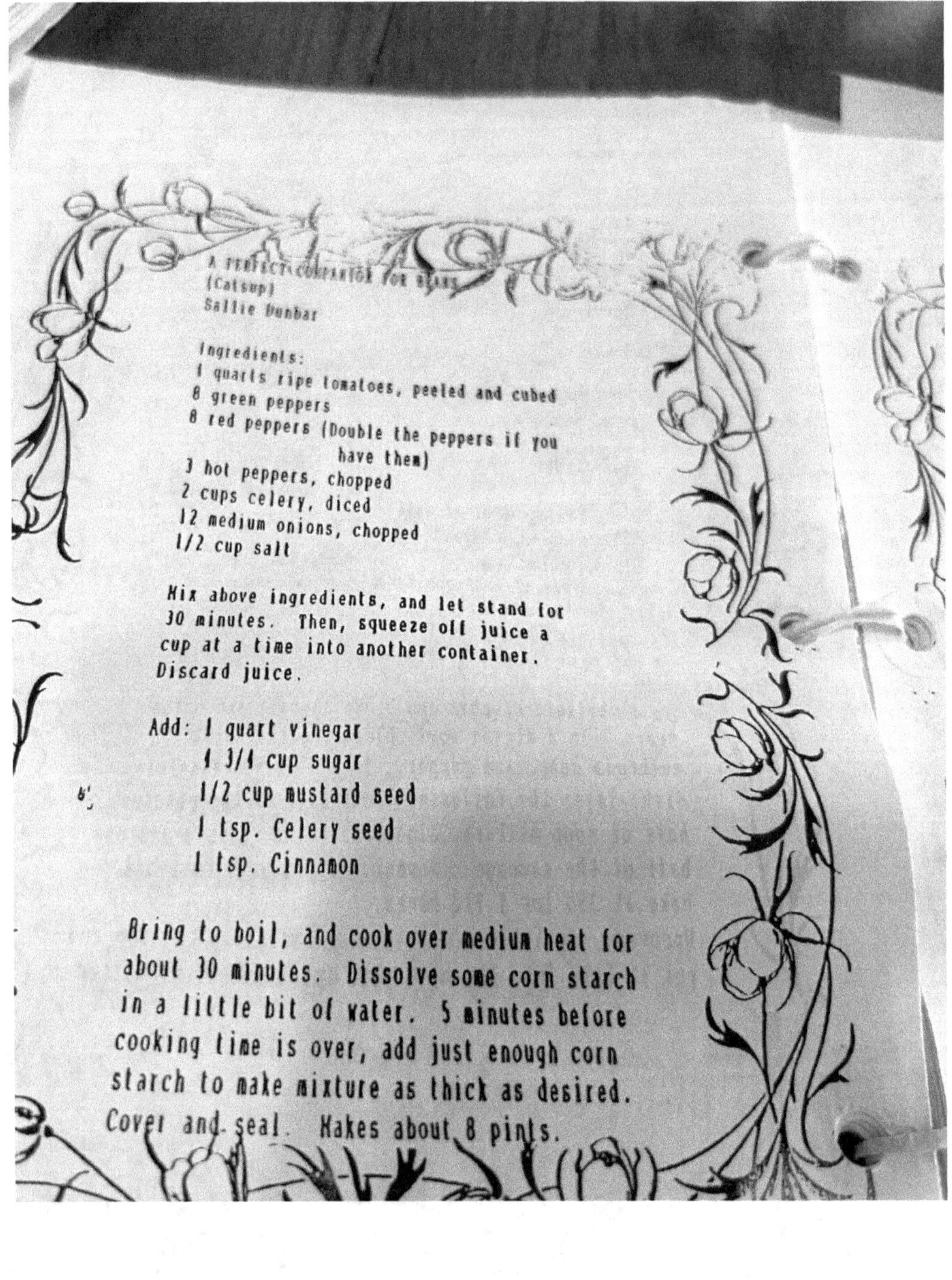

A PERFECT COMPANION FOR BEANS
(Catsup)
Sallie Dunbar

Ingredients:
1 quarts ripe tomatoes, peeled and cubed
8 green peppers
8 red peppers (Double the peppers if you
                have them)
3 hot peppers, chopped
2 cups celery, diced
12 medium onions, chopped
1/2 cup salt

Mix above ingredients, and let stand for
30 minutes. Then, squeeze off juice a
cup at a time into another container.
Discard juice.

Add: 1 quart vinegar
     1 3/4 cup sugar
     1/2 cup mustard seed
     1 tsp. Celery seed
     1 tsp. Cinnamon

Bring to boil, and cook over medium heat for
about 30 minutes. Dissolve some corn starch
in a little bit of water. 5 minutes before
cooking time is over, add just enough corn
starch to make mixture as thick as desired.
Cover and seal. Makes about 8 pints.

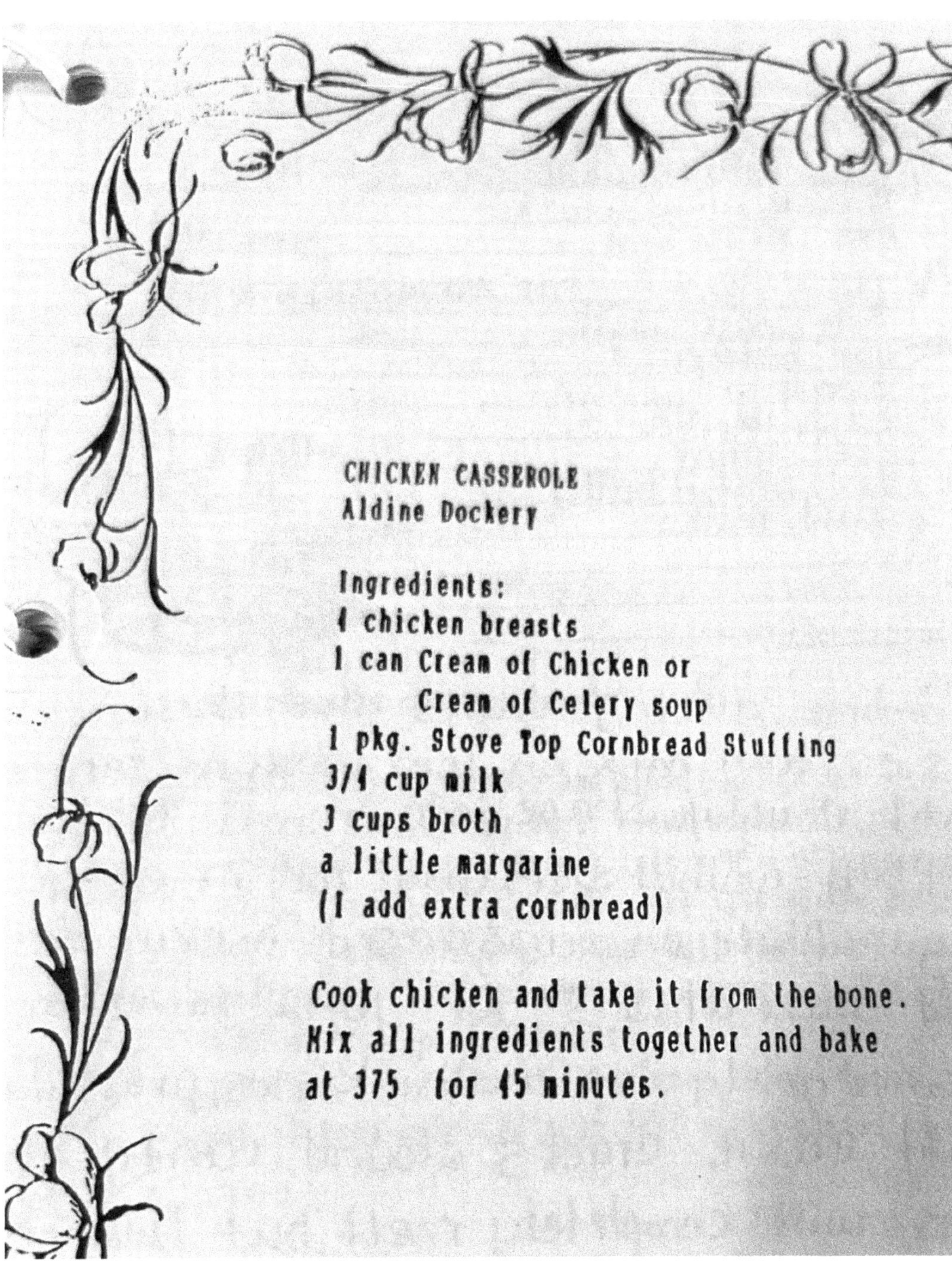

CHICKEN CASSEROLE
Aldine Dockery

Ingredients:
4 chicken breasts
1 can Cream of Chicken or
        Cream of Celery soup
1 pkg. Stove Top Cornbread Stuffing
3/4 cup milk
3 cups broth
a little margarine
(I add extra cornbread)

Cook chicken and take it from the bone.
Mix all ingredients together and bake
at 375 for 45 minutes.

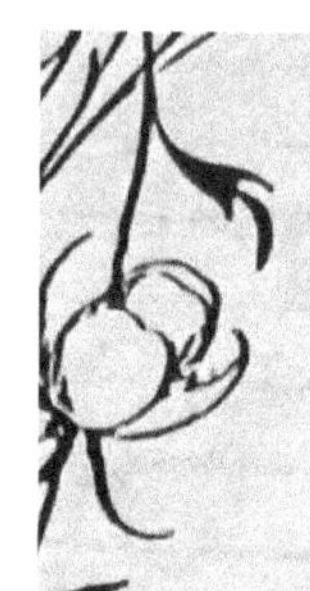

Turtle Cake
Brenda Bault

1 box German Chocolate Cake Mix
1 14 oz. bag caramels (48)
1 stick butter
1/3 cup evaporated milk
1 cup chocolate chips
1 cup of chopped nuts

Mix cake mix according to directions. Pour half of batter into greased 9 x 13 pan. Bake at 350 degrees for 15 minutes. In pan over low heat, melt caramels, butter, and milk. Remover cake from oven, pour caramel mixture over cake. Sprinkle with chocolate chips and pecans.

Add remaining half of batter. Bake at 350 degrees for 20 minutes.

Recipe: Coconut Supreme Cake
From: Thelma Basil
Makes: ______

1 pkg. White or Yellow Cake Mix
1 (4 serving size) Jell-O Vanilla
    instant pudding
1 1/3 C. Water
4 eggs
1/4 C. oil
2 C. Flake Coconut
1 C. Chopped Pecans

Blend Cake Mix, Pudding, Water, eggs and oil in large mixing bowl. Beat at medium speed 4 Minutes. Stir in coconut and nuts. Pour into 3 (9 inch) layer pans, greased and floured. Bake at 350° for 35 M.

Coconut Supreme Frosting

4 Tbsp. Butter or Margarine
2 C. Coconut   1/2 tsp. Vanilla
1 (8 oz.) Cream Cheese   2 tsp. milk
3 1/2 C. Confectioners Sugar

Melt just 2 tablespoons Butter in skillet. add 1/4 cups Coconut. Stir over low heat until golden brown. Spread on paper towel to cool. Cream 2 tablespoons butter with Cream Cheese. add milk. Beat in sugar. blend in Vanilla and 1 3/4 cups Cocon. Spread on each cake layer

Lazy Peach Cobbler
Michelle Kerr

1/2 cup butter
1 cup flour
1 cup sugar
1 egg
3/4 cup milk
2 cans peaches in heavy syrup
1 tsp. vanilla

Melt butter in casserole pan.
Mix flour, sugar, egg, and
milk together. Pour over
butter. Add vanilla to
peaches with syrup and pour
over top of batter. Do not
stir. Bake at 350 degrees for
1 hour.

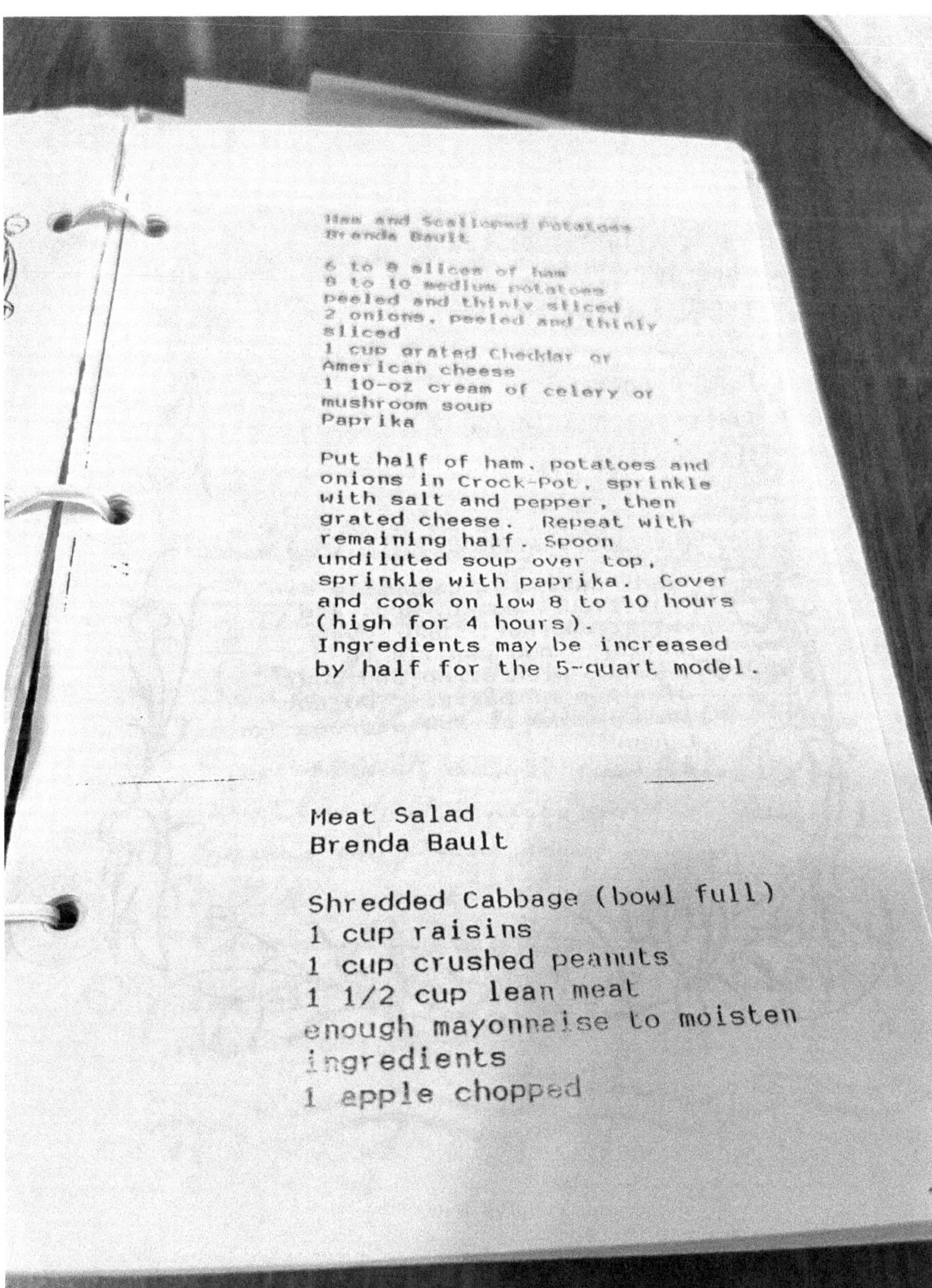

Ham and Scalloped Potatoes
Brenda Bault

6 to 8 slices of ham
8 to 10 medium potatoes
peeled and thinly sliced
2 onions, peeled and thinly
sliced
1 cup grated Cheddar or
American cheese
1 10-oz cream of celery or
mushroom soup
Paprika

Put half of ham, potatoes and
onions in Crock-Pot, sprinkle
with salt and pepper, then
grated cheese. Repeat with
remaining half. Spoon
undiluted soup over top,
sprinkle with paprika. Cover
and cook on low 8 to 10 hours
(high for 4 hours).
Ingredients may be increased
by half for the 5-quart model.

Meat Salad
Brenda Bault

Shredded Cabbage (bowl full)
1 cup raisins
1 cup crushed peanuts
1 1/2 cup lean meat
enough mayonnaise to moisten
ingredients
1 apple chopped

PEACH CAKE
Jane Johnson

2 eggs, slightly beaten
2 cups sugar
2 cups self rising flour
1 tsp. soda
1 tsp. cinnamon
1 quart peaches (chopped)
1 stick margarine

Beat eggs, then add other ingredients.
Bake at 350 for 30 minutes.

Topping:
Mix: 1/2 cup sugar
      1/2 cup evaporated milk
      1 stick margarine
      1 tsp. vanilla

Cook 5 minutes, then pour over warm cake.

CONGEALED SALAD
Aldine Dockery

Ingredients:

1 small can crushed pineapple
3/4 cup water
1 pkg. jello (any flavor)
1 medium apple (cubed)
1 medium banana (sliced)
1/2 cup pecans, optional
1 small container of Cool Whip

Mix pineapple, jello, and water and bring
to boil.
Cool till jello begins to gel. Add apple,
banana, and pecans. Fold in the Cool Whip.
Rub mold or dish with margarine to keep
salad from sticking. Fill. Chill until firm.

Potato Sausage Casserole
By Cassie McGowan

1 lb. sausage
1 can cheddar cheese soup
Boiled potatoes (salted and
cubed
1/2 c. milk

Boil and drain potatoes. Fry
and drain sausage. Mix
cheddar cheese soup, milk, and
sausage. Simmer to melt soup.
Add mixture to drained
potatoes in a casserole dish.
Bake 30 minutes at 350
degrees.

Chocolate Fudge Candy
Renda Johnson

4 1/2 cups sugar
2 sticks margarine
1/4 cup white syrup
1 can carnation milk
Cook 12 minutes
Add 1 package of chocolate
chips.

Cinnamon Ring Pickles
Renda Johnson

Peel and cut out seeds
1 Gallon Pickles
1 cup lime
4 1/2 quarts water

Put rings in lime water. Let
stand 24 hours. Drain wash in
cold water. Then: Soak in
fresh cold water 3 hrs. Drain.
Mix 1/2 cup vinegar
1 bottle red food color
1 tablespoon alum
Enough water to cover pickles.
Heat and simmer 2 hrs. Drain.

Syrup
1 cup vinegar
1 cup water
5 cups sugar
4 sticks cinnamon
1/2 bag cinn. candy (Red Hots)
Bring to a boil, pour over
pickles for 3 mornings then
can. Double to make more.

Broccoli Casserole
By Cassie McGowan

1 c. celery chopped
1/2 c. onion chopped
2 T. butter
1 can cream of mushroom soup
1 can cream of chicken soup
1 18 oz. Cheese Whiz
1 pkg. chopped broccoli cooked
as directed and drained
1 c. cooked rice

Saute celery and onion in
butter. Combine soups and
cheese whiz in pan, heat until
well blended. Combine
broccoli, onion mixture, soups
and rive. Pour into 8 x 10
casserole. Sprinkle with
paprika. Bake at 375 degrees
10 minutes.

Sweet Potato Pie
By Zillie Luttrel

9 med. sweet potatoes
Boil until done and peel
Add: 2 sticks butter and mash
1/2 c. brown sugar
1/2 c. white sugar
1/2 t. salt
1/4 t. nutmeg
2 c. milk
3 eggs

Makes 2 pies. Bake at 350
degrees until done. You may
put marshmallows on top and
broil.

Pork Chops and Potatoes
By ... Potatoes?

4 to 8 pork chops (boneless)
1 onion (sliced)
2 lb. ... of potatoes
Salt (to taste)
Pepper (to taste)
1 can cream of chicken soup
1/2 can water

Brown pork chops on both sides
and put in bottom of baking
dish, cover with sliced
onions, slice potatoes and
layer them, with the salt and
pepper on each layer. fill the
baking dish, then add 2 t. of
bacon drippings on top of the
potatoes. Then add the can of
cream of chicken soup with the
water   Sprinkle pepper on top
of that and bake at 400
degrees for an hour or until
the potatoes are tender.
(These are good with other
meats or you can use your
favorite soup).

Potato Casserole
By Barbara Wilson

Potatoes (salted) cooked and
drained
1 can cheddar cheese soup
1/2 cup milk
1 lb. sausage (mild or hot)

Brown sausage. drain fat. Mix
soup, milk, and sausage. Pour
over potatoes in a baking
dish. Bake 30 minutes in oven
at 400 degrees.
(If uncooked potatoes, bake 1
hour, 15 minutes.)

Fruit Salad
By Cassie McGowan

2 cans chunk pineapple (save
juice)
2 cans chunk fruit (drained)
1 can mandarin oranges
(drained)
3 bananas, sliced

Take pineapple juice, add 1
box instant vanilla pudding, 3
tablespoons of Tang Mix with
fruit.

Corn Bread Salad
By Betty Popplewell

1 green pepper, diced
2 tomatoes, diced
1 sweet onion, diced
6 eggs boiled & diced
1 lb. bacon, fried crisp,
crumbled
1 large pone of cornbread,
(crumbled)
mayonnaise or salad dressing

In a large bowl, mix together
ingredients with enough
mayonnaise to make mixture
moist (it should stick
together). Allow to stand
over night in refrigerator in
covered dish.

Chili Bake
By Avalene Dockery

Make your favorite chili, or
if you have some left over.
Put chili in casserole dish,
add 1 can whole kernel corn,
then mix in mixing bowl about
2 cups corn meal a little
flour and milk just like you
would if making cornbread.
Then drop by spoonfuls on top
of chili. Bake at 400 degrees
until cornbread is brown.

Chicken & Noodles
By Charolette Leis

1 c. boneless chicken (cooked
done)
1 can cream of chicken soup
2 pkgs. of chicken gravy mix
12 oz. water
10 oz. milk
1 large bag egg noodles

Boil egg noodles 'til done &
drain. Mix remaining
ingredients well and ass to
egg noodles. Cook over medium
heat about 10 minutes.

Deer BBQ
By Charolette Leis

Cook 5 lbs. deer roast & 1
large onion chopped, cook
until tender.

Drain and shred roast and add
2 bottles of Kraft Thick and
Spicy Honey Barbecue. Let
simmer and serve.

Seven Layer Salad
By Avalene Dockery

1 c. cauliflower, chopped
1 c. celery, chopped
1 c. green onions, chopped
1 pkg. frozen green peas,
thawed and drained,
1 c. mayonnaise
1 pkg. cheddar cheese grated
7 strips bacon fried, crisp
and crumbled.

Place alternating layers of
vegetables in bowl spread
mayonnaise over top. Cover
with grated cheese and bacon.
Garnish with olives if
desired, will keep in
refrigerator for about one
week.

Earlene's Peach Treat

2 - 3z. boxes Peach Jello
(Mix according to directions)
    Let begin to jell

Then add —

1 cup Coconut
1 8z. can Crushed pineapple (drained)
2 bananas (sliced)
1 cup Miniature Marshmallows
mix with jello & pour into dish & chill.

Topping —

Cook together over low heat —
1 cup sugar
1 lg. tablespoon Cornstarch or Flour
1 egg, beaten
1 tablespoon butter
Juice from pineapple —
When thick beat in 8z Cream Cheese
            Let Cool

Add 1 - 8z. Carton Cool Whip —

Spread over jello Mixture

"Salmon Loaf"
(microwave)

2 - Cans (15½ oz) salmon
1 - cup dry bread crumbs
2 - eggs beaten
2 - TBSp lemon juice
½ - tsp. salt
1 - TBSP. instant minced onions
1 - TBSP. dried parsley flakes
¼ - tsp. pepper

Drain salmon reserving liquid, mash bones. Add
enough milk to reserved salmon liquid to make
1 cup. Mix thoroughly with remaining ingredient.
Pour into dish 9 x 5 inches. Microwave at high
until center is set 7 to 11 minutes. Rotate loaf
Let stand 5 minutes.

Million Dollar Rice Salad

1 large pkg marshmallows (diced)
1 large can crushed pineapple (drained)
1 8 oz pkg cream cheese
2 tbsp. sugar
1 tbsp. mayonnaise
2 cup cooked rice
12 or more maraschino cherries
1 cup whipping cream, whipped or cool whip.
Pecans if desired

Cut marshmallows in small pieces Add
drained pineapple, cream the cheese
sugar and mayonnaise until smooth
Add rice, cherries & marshmallows
Mix, fold in whipped cream & nuts,
Chill before serving.

Colletti's Cocoa Cake

3/4 cup butter or margarine
1 3/4. cups sugar
2 eggs
1 teaspoon vanilla
2 cups unsifted all purpose flour
3/4 cup cocoa
1 1/4 teaspoon baking soda
1/2 teaspoon salt
1 1/3 cups water

Cream butter or margarine and sugar until
light & fluffy. Add eggs and vanilla, beat
1 minute at medium speed. Combine
cocoa, baking soda and salt, add alt.
with water to creamed mixture. Pour
batter into 2 pans (greased) and floured.
Bake at 350° 35 to 40 minutes for
or for 9 inch pans 30 to 35 minutes
& frost.

PEANUT CLUSTERS

1 cup chocolate chips
1/2 cup peanut butter (chunky or
  creamy)
1 cup salted peanuts

Melt chocolate chips and peanut butter over very low heat. Stir to prevent sticking. Add peanuts and stir well until all peanuts are coated with chocolate. Drop by teaspoonfuls on waxed paper. Chill until firm.

BUTTERSCOTCH PEANUT BUTTER CANDY BALLS

2 lbs. confectioners sugar
3 sticks margarine
1 (12 oz.) jar crunchy Peter Pan peanut butter
¾ stick paraffin
2 pkgs. butterscotch chips (small)

STEP 1

Melt paraffin in double boiler and add butterscotch chips. Mix well. Keep on low heat while dipping candy balls.

STEP II

Melt margarine on low heat. Pour into confectioner sugar. Mix well, add peanut butter and mix well. Make into balls and dip into butterscotch chips mixture. After dipped put on greased sheet.

Guess What Cake

6 egg whites (stiffly beaten)
2 cups sugar
2 tsp. vanilla
1 cup chopped nuts
50 to 60 Ritz Crackers (coarsely broken)

Mix and bake in oblong pan at
350° for 30 min

2 pkg Dream Whip - mix according to
8 oz. pkg. Cream Cheese
1 Can Crushed pineapple (about 15 oz)
Mix and spread over crust
(Best if made a day before serving and
refrigerate

"No Egg Banana Pudding"

3 boxes Vanilla or French Vanilla instant pudding
3 - cups cold milk
1 - large Cool Whip (16 oz)
About 6 banana's (as many as you like)
Vanilla wafer's (about 1½ box's) (Graham Crackers can be used)
1 - Small Sour Cream (optional)

Wip instant pudding with milk, @ low speed on Mixer.
Stir in Cool Whip & Sour cream. Then layer
banana's & vanilla wafers in container.
Lay a few vanilla wafers on top for
decoration or sprinkle vanilla wafer
crumbs on the top.

"Corn Chip Salad"

2 - Cans Whole Kernel Corn (drained)
½ - red onion (Chopped)
1 - Bell Pepper (Chopped)
2 - Cups shredded Cheddar Cheese
1 - cup mayo or salad dressing
1 - Bag Chili Cheese Frito Corn Chips

Mix all ingredients together. (except Chips)
Add Frito Chips before serving.

Very Berry Salad
By Modine Vaught

2 pkgs. Raspberry Jello
1 c. boiling water
1 can cherry pie filling
1 can crushed pineapple (do
not drain)

Mix in order listed, pour in
dish and let set until firm.

Mix: 8 oz cream cheese
(softened)
1 t. vanilla
1 c. sour cream

Spread over jello mixture
(that has set) Sprinkle with
1/2 c. chopped English
walnuts.

You can also use Blue Berry
Pie Filling. I even used
whole Cranberry Sauce. Make
this for diabetics: use sugar
free jello, low-fat cream
cheese, low fat sour cream
sugar free fruit or light.

Watergate Salad
By Tonva Coffey

1 Box Pastico pudding
(instant)
1 9 oz. Cool Whip
1 c. miniature marshmallows
1 c. chopped nuts
1 20 oz. crushed pineapple
with juice.

Mix pudding in pineapple with
juice   Add cool whip- add
marshmallows and nuts. Ready
to serve.

Strawberry Pie
By Debra Wilson

1 pint strawberries
1 c. sugar
4 T. flour
1 pkg. Strawberry Jello

Dissolve sugar, flour, and
jello together in 1 cup of
boiling water, let come to a
boil (kind of thick). Set off
and cool. drain strawberries
then place in crust, pour
mixture over top of
strawberries. Makes one pie.

Christmas Punch
By Tonya Coffey

1 can red Hawaiian Punch
1 pkg. punch Kool-aid with 1
c. sugar
1 quart Ginger Ale
1 small can frozen lemonade
plus 3 cans water.

Mix well and chill.

Corn Pudding
By Debra Wilson

3 eggs
4 T. sugar
1 T. flour (heaping)
1 T. salt
1 pkg. frozen corn or 2 1/2 c.
fresh corn or 2 cans drained
1 c. milk
Pinch of baking powder

Beat eggs. Add flour, baking
powder and salt to sugar and
stir into eggs. Add fresh or
partially thawed corn and
milk. Pour into a butter
baking dish and dot with small
pieces of butter. Bake in
oven at 325 degrees for about
1 hour or until firm.

Cauliflower Salad
By Modine Vaught

1 med. head of cabbage-
shredded, shave don't grate
1 med. head cauliflower also
shaved, or sliced thin
1 lb. bacon-fried crisp and
cut up
1/4 cup sugar
1/3 cup Parmesan cheese
1 cup mayonnaise
1 med onion

Mix ingredients together in
order given and refrigerate-
at least 2 hrs.

Sensational Double Layer
Pumpkin Pie
By Modine Vaught

4 oz. Cream cheese, softened
1 T. milk or half & half
1 T. sugar
1 1/2 C. thawed cool whip
1 Graham cracker Pie crust
1 C. cold milk or half & half
2 pkgs. (4 oz) Jello-Vanilla
Instant Pudding
1 can (16 oz.) pumpkin
1 t. ground cinnamon
1/2 t. ginger
1/4 t. cloves

Mix cream cheese, 1 T. mild &
sugar in large bowl with wire
whisk until smooth. Gently
stir in whipped topping.
Spread on crust.

Pour 1 C. milk into bowl. Add
pudding mix. Beat with wire
whisk until well blended, (1-2
min) will be thick.

Stir in pumpkin & spices. Mix
well, spread over cream cheese
layer. Refrigerate at lest 3
hrs. Garnish with additional
whipped topping and a sprinkle
of nuts if you desire.

P.S. I made this with low fat
cream cheese, skim milk and
sweetener plus sugar free
jello pudding. I, also, put
this in regular pie crust.

Glen Lane's Chicken Salad
Submitted by Sallie C. Dunbar

4 cups chopped, cooked chicken
or (tuna)
1 cup chopped celery
1/2 cup chopped sweet pickles
2 cups seedless white grapes-
halved
3/4 cup chopped pecans
1 cup sour cream
1 cup mayonnaise
4 hard boiled eggs (chopped)
1 tsp salt

Combine all ingredients, toss
lightly. Chill 2 hours.
Serve on lettuce with crackers
of any kind.

Dr. Pepper Chili

2 lbs. ground beef(or ground
chuck), browned and drained
1/2 c. chopped onion
1/8 t. garlic Power
2 t. salt
1/8 t. oregano
1 t. black pepper
1 T. paprika
6 oz. c. tomato paste
2 cups or 1 can Dr. Pepper
1 1/4 cups water
chili powder to taste.

Bring all to boil, Simmer at
least 1 hour to blend flavors.

Neiman Marcus Cake

1st layer
1 Swiss Chocolate Cake Mix
2 eggs
1 c. pecans
1 stick melted butter
Grease 9 x 13 pan, spread. It
will be very thick.

2nd layer
8 oz. cream cheese (softened)
1 lb. powdered sugar
2 eggs
1 t. vanilla
Beat and spread on top of 1st
layer. Bake 350 degrees for
45 minutes. Cool.
Topping (optional)
8 oz. cool whip
1/2 c. of coconut
1/2 c. pecans
grated Hershey

I use Butter Pecan Cake mix
and leave off topping for a
great change.

Biscuits

2 c. self-rising flour
¼ c. vegetable shortening
¾ c. milk

Heat oven to 450'F

Place flour in large bowl. Cut in shortening with pastry blender until crumbs are the size of peas. Add milk, stirring with fork until soft dough forms.

Turn dough onto lightly floured surface. Knead gently 5 to 6 times, just until smooth.

Rollout dough to ½ inch thickness.

Cut with floured 2 inch round cutter.

Arrange on baking sheet with sides touching.

Bake 10 to 12 minutes or until golden brown.

Serve warm.
Makes 1 dozen

White Bean and Chicken Chili

This bean and chicken-filled chili is a rich source of fiber and protein.
Stir in the chopped cooked chicken at the end of cooking to keep the
Chicken most. Serve topped with a spoonful of salsa and chopped cilantro.

1 t. Olive oil
1 med. Onion, chopped
4 cloves of garlic
2 t. Ground cumin
1 t. Dried oregano
½ cup chopped green chilies
3 cups Great Northern beans
4 cups chicken broth
4 cups diced cooked chicken breast
¼ cup of salsa
¼ cup of chopped fresh cilantro

In a soup pot, heat the olive oil over medium heat. Add the onion and cook
until softened, about 5 min. Stir in garlic, cumin, and oregano, and cook
for about 1 min. Add green chilies, beans and broth. Bring to boil, reduce
Heat to a simmer, and cook for about 20 min. Stir in chicken and cook
For about 10 more min. Now it is done.

Buttercream Frosting

½ c. (1 stick) butter at room temperature
½ c. vegetable shortening
4 c. powered sugar
1 tsp. vanilla extract
1-2 Tbsp Water

Directions:
In a mixing bowl, beat together butter and shortening.
add powered sugar to butter mixture one cup at a
time. Make sure each cup of sugar is well incorporated
before adding the next cup. Beat in vanilla. Add 1-2
tablespoon of water until desired consistency is reached.